S0-CIF-894

MAN AT HIS BEST

MAN AT HIS BEST

How to Be More Youthful, Virile, Healthy, and Handsome

RUSSELL L. RHODES

Illustrated by Eduardo Valdes

Photographs by Klaus Lucka

DOUBLEDAY & COMPANY, INC., GARDEN CITY, NEW YORK

ISBN: 0-385-05906-x
Library of Congress Catalog Card Number 73–22791

Printed in the United States of America

Dedicated to Dusty Rhodes
and all other men
who have the desire
to lead a happy and successful life.

I wish to acknowledge and thank these organizations and people as well as the many others who have given me their co-operation and help in writing this book:

Colgate-Palmolive Ltd.
Clairol, Inc.
Energen Foods Company
Fabergé Incorporated
Hand & Nail Culture Institute Ltd.
Michaeljohn
Planned Parenthood Federation of America, Inc.
Scholl (U.K.) Ltd.
Wella (Gt. Britain) Ltd.
World Health Organization, Geneva

Edwin H. S. Alcock, B.D.S. (New Zealand)
Vincent M. Cali, D.D.S.
Michael N. Landon, M.I.T. (London) A.R.I.P.H.H.
Robert H. Newman, M.D.
P. G. F. Nixon, F.R.C.P.
Alistair Murray, M.S.R.G.
Kenneth Tomlinson, B.Sc., B.A., F.R.I.C.
J. G. P. Williams, F.R.C.S., D.Phys.Med.

Contents

Introduction

Let's face it: Every man among us would like to be more handsome and in better physical condition. It's not only a natural desire, but by today's standards, it's essential.

Unfair as it may seem, more and more studies show that in business, given two men of equal ability, the better-looking one usually gets the better job. Last year while driving to a conference in Cannes, the president of a major international service organization confided to me that one of the reasons for the rapid growth of his company was his policy to promote only attractive men to the important positions involving direct personal contact with the company's clients. The less attractive men were kept under wraps doing the donkey work. "After all," he said, "most people prefer to associate and work with good-looking men. Right or wrong, I give my clients what makes them happy."

Aside from business success, a successful and happy social life also depends a great deal on a good-looking appearance and a youthful spirit. Handsome men don't stand on the sidelines; they're in the swing of things enjoying the good life. Fit men don't waste time pampering weak backs and hearts; they're where the action is, having fun. And don't underestimate the effect your looks and physical condition have on your sex life: they can most certainly improve it.

Most men can benefit from this book in one way or another. It can help make you more handsome, feel younger and fitter, and give you a slimmer, healthier body within just thirty days. It can show you how to shed years from your appearance and increase your virility, or how to deal more effectively with the stresses inherent in a successful business career. In short, it will help you live a happier and more productive life.

For over fifteen years I've had frank discussions with chemists and researchers who have shown me the subtleties of the human body and how it reacts to various preparations, exercises, and diets. This book contains the secrets of some of the largest American and European manufacturers who develop every conceivable type of grooming, toiletry, and cosmetic preparation to make men and women more beautiful. It contains advice from top Olympic coaches, doctors, heart specialists, and nutritionists. Dynamic "jet set" tycoons from all over the world and theater people, whose fame and fortunes depend upon their continuing good looks, have confided their tips on how they hold on to youth and make themselves more handsome. Thus this is a practical book. It's a handbook designed to help you become better looking, healthier, and more fit with a minimum of effort.

Don't feel funny or embarrassed about this subject or any of the methods this book recommends for improving your looks and fitness. Isn't it only common sense to make yourself more attractive to compete more successfully in your business career? Isn't it logical that as science works to prolong your life, you should work to prolong your youthful vitality and your ability to enjoy the extra years to the fullest? When you look in the mirror or get out on the beach, do you feel nature has dealt you a few cards from the bottom of the pack? If so, here's your chance to get a reshuffle.

CHAPTER I

Your First Step to Better Looks and Fitness

Just reading this book can be of great importance to your overall health and appearance. It will define and make you aware of problem areas that you may now be overlooking or will face in the future. But I hope you won't be satisfied with just being aware of these problems. I hope you'll use this book critically and positively to achieve dramatic improvements in your looks, health and fitness. With relatively little effort you should start seeing results within thirty days.

As your first step, take a hard, honest look in the mirror and commit yourself to improving what you see. Analyze your appearance feature by feature, head to toe, starting with your hair and working down (the book has been arranged in this order). Also analyze your health. Do you live under business or emotional tension, have cholesterol and weight problems, or lack energy?

Compare each part of your body to the criteria for perfection listed in the book. Compare your mental outlook as well. Select those areas that you feel most need improving and those that you should protect against aging. Then pull together the recommended regimens which will improve and protect them. Remember to set realistic goals for yourself, and keep things simple. Your combined regimens must be comfortable and easy to follow so they'll become a pleasant and natural part of your daily routine.

The younger "Mr. Perfects" who read this book may have to make only small changes in their appearance, because physically they have little that needs improving—at the present time. But if they take preventative action now to maintain their appearance and start training their minds to control stress, they should enjoy their youthful good looks for years to come.

The rest of you men should expect much greater improvement in your looks, health, and fitness. The degree depends upon what nature gave you to start with, the amount of neglect to your body that you must correct, and the stresses under which you're working. I'm sure you'll be surprised how much better you can look and feel merely by changing a few grooming habits and learning how to relax. Theory is fine, but if you want some of the advantages that your better-looking contemporaries enjoy, you'd better get off your butt and start.

CHAPTER 2

Hair: How to Improve and Keep an Attractive Head of Hair

When you think that hair is the most visible and controllable feature of one's appearance, it's no wonder men spend so much time, thought, and money on it—probably more than on any other part of their body. During his lifetime the average man will spend between five and eight thousand dollars on having his hair cut, shampooing it, and buying lotions. But money alone won't achieve good-looking hair.

One thing all men have in common: we don't want to lose our hair. Lots of factors affect its health and vitality, and you should know what they are. Some have been magnified out of all proportion and probably have little importance for you; but others need your constant attention. By following the regimen recommended by this book, you should be able to improve the appearance of your hair and keep it healthy. After all, your alternative isn't very pleasant. Dirty, neglected hair and dandruff may reward you later on with ugly scalp problems and baldness.

YOUR GOAL: THE PERFECT HEAD OF HAIR

The perfect head of hair is a full head of hair with little, if any, recession. The hair is clean, with a natural sheen and enough body so you can comb and style it any way you like. It isn't too porous and doesn't have broken or split ends. Your scalp should be free of excess oil, loose scale, and all irritation. In fact, you shouldn't be aware of your scalp at all. Your hair should fall neatly into place and be styled to blend naturally with your over-all appearance. It flatters *you,* without drawing attention to *itself.*

IMPROVE THE CONDITION OF YOUR HAIR

First, keep it clean

The most important thing you can do to keep your hair and maintain its health is to make sure it's clean at all times. Very few men do this, much to their future sorrow. Next, as the vitality of your hair and health of your scalp depend a lot on your physical and mental health, stick to a balanced diet, have regular physical checkups, and learn to relax.

How often should you wash your hair?

As a general rule, wash **oily hair** at least every two or three days in tepid water; wash a **very dry scalp** and hair about every five days in warmer water to stimulate oil production. Environmental conditions and internal body changes affect the amount of oil your scalp produces, so you may have to wash your hair more or less to suit conditions.

Of course the dirtier your job conditions and the greater the air pollution from smoke, chemical waste, etc., the more often you need to shampoo. But don't worry. Oily hair can be washed as often as once a day. Unless a scalp is extremely dry or suffers some problem condition, hair can seldom be hurt from too much washing.

Apply your shampoo twice and work it through the hair onto your scalp gently, but thoroughly. If you rub too hard, you can injure wet hair. Don't expect much lather from the first application, but the second one should give you a good lather to show you've used enough. Too much lather, particulary at the start, will neither help nor harm your hair—it's just wasteful. Rinse well after each application to completely remove all shampoo and dirt.

Use the right shampoo for your hair and scalp

The main purpose of a shampoo is to clean, so today most shampoos contain detergents that remove dirt and oil effectively in all water conditions. Unless your doctor recommends it, don't wash your hair with soap. When used in hard water, it will leave a dull scum on the hair.

Choose a shampoo designed for the degree of oiliness of your hair, its texture (fine or coarse), and the condition of your scalp. Don't just pick up the first one you see or one you recall from advertising. Read package directions carefully. Too strong a shampoo can strip your scalp of too much oil, leaving it dry and itchy. A very mild one may not be strong enough to clean oily hair well. (If you're not sure about the degree of oiliness of your scalp and the texture and condition of your hair, ask your barber.) Shampoos also come in a wide variety of medicated formulations containing tars, sulfur compounds, and bacteriostats to treat dandruff and other scalp problems. Use them on the recommendation of your doctor or a qualified pharmacist, not the advice of some satisfied friend who may have quite a different scalp condition from yours.

Condition difficult hair to improve its appearance

If your hair gives you trouble because of its fine texture, is flyaway, or has become porous and coarse from overexposure to the sun and wind, try applying a conditioner to it every week or so.

Conditioners are adsorbed onto the surface of your hair, giving it additional body and making it more supple for easier combing and control. They also leave hair with a smooth feel and finish.

Conditioners are made for every type of hair texture and degree of oiliness. You usually apply them after a shampoo, wait several minutes, and rinse them out. They can often last through several shampooings. Some shampoos contain their own built-in conditioners.

Throw away your hairbrush!

This may come as a shock to you, but most experts consider brushing one of the worst things you can do to your hair. All that brushing done by Scarlet O'Hara didn't improve the quality and luster of her hair; it merely pulled it, twisted it, and split its ends. The same thing applies to men.

Use a brush gently and sparingly at night *only* to remove any dust and loose dirt which may have accumulated on it during the day. Don't use it when your hair is wet and in its most vulnerable state. Better still, don't use it at all. But if you can't break years of habit, at least keep the damage to a minimum. Make sure your brush has natural or well-rounded nylon bristles and keep it, and your comb, clean.

Should you massage your scalp?

There's nothing inherently bad about massage if done well. Unfortunately, most men end up massaging their hair, not their scalp. Rubbing your hair back and forth under pressure can damage it, and besides, your scalp normally gets enough massage from regular shampooing.

If your doctor, dermatologist, or a qualified trichologist insists on massage for your particular scalp condition, do it gently. Put your fingers through your hair to the scalp and use the tips to carefully move the scalp, not the hair, back and forth. Don't let your fingertips slide over your scalp. Start your massage at the nape of your neck and your temples and work toward the crown of your head.

Watch out for possible scalp disease

Keep an eye open for any symptoms like an itchy or inflamed scalp, a visible increase in its oil production, and uncontrollable dandruff or scaling. If unchecked, some scalp conditions can lead to hair degeneration and baldness. When correctly diagnosed and caught in the early stages, most of these conditions can be cured, or at least serious problems prevented. Consult an expert at the first sign of trouble.

Treat dandruff; don't let it go unchecked

Your scalp normally sheds some skin tissue, or scale, at a relatively constant rate. There's no harm in this. Dandruff is also skin tissue, but tissue produced and shed in greater than normal quantities. It's the sign of a bad scalp condition which, if left untreated, can lead to more serious complications.

Dandruff attacks dry, normal, and oily scalps and is common among young men, usually tapering off in middle age. It starts when the sebaceous glands in the scalp receive increased hormone stimulation and step up their oil production. (You may not always notice this on a dry scalp.) The bacteria living on the scalp adapt themselves and flourish in this new, oil-rich environment, stimulating the glands to produce even greater quantities of oil. A vicious cycle develops which causes the scalp to make abnormally high amounts of skin tissue which it sloughs off in the form we call dandruff.

Nervousness, spicy foods, alcohol, and other things that increase blood circulation and stimulate the oil glands can aggravate this condition. Itching, possibly with some inflammation, usually accompanies dandruff.

Treat dandruff by cleaning excess oil and scale from your scalp and applying a bacteriostat to discourage bacteria growth. You can buy many medicated formulations and dandruff shampoos combining both cleaning agents and bacteriostats. Make sure you get the one best suited to your scalp condition and hair type. Ask your doctor or pharmacist for advice. Finally, remove secondary aggravating factors where possible.

AVOID THINGS THAT HARM YOUR HAIR

Sun is good for your scalp and hair in small doses, but overexposure can dry them and make your hair porous and feel harsh. Dark hair can take more sun than blond, but in hot climates, all of us should protect our hair from the really fierce summer sun between noon and four in the afternoon. Remember to take into account the sun's drying effects when deciding what strength shampoo to take on your vacation.

Chlorine water in pools doesn't actually harm your hair or scalp, but if left on hair exposed to lots of sunlight, the chlorine tends to bleach it. This streaked, outdoor effect may be very flattering to you—it certainly marks you as an athlete. After large doses of chlorine and sun, very light hair often picks up a greenish tinge. **Salt water** is good for your scalp, but it dulls your hair and makes it sticky and difficult to comb. You'd best rinse it out before leaving the beach. **Hard water** doesn't harm hair, contrary to what many people think. As mentioned earlier, when used with soap, it leaves a dulling film on hair. Don't use too much water, hard or soft, when combing you hair because it removes some natural oil and can leave hair looking dull.

Avoid diet extremes. When I asked an expert from an international cosmetic house about the effects of diet on hair, he blew his stack. Beating a fist on the table, he exploded that "there's too much talk about the harmful effects of a poor diet on hair and too many beauty writers use it to scare readers." He explained that over 95 per cent of all men living in North America, Britain, and northern Europe eat well enough to get everything their bodies need for healthy hair. Unless some part of your system isn't functioning properly, you shouldn't need vitamin or mineral supplements.

If by some chance you *did* have a dietary deficiency severe enough to make a noticeable difference in the condition of your hair, you wouldn't be worrying about your hair—you'd be too busy running from doctor to doctor trying to cure all the other far more serious problems erupting throughout your entire body.

One word of warning, however. Be careful of crash diets. Some throw your system out of balance and can deprive it of proper nourishment. These have been known to make hair dull, brittle, and lifeless and, in extreme cases, have caused some hair loss.

Disease and illnesses which sap strength from your body also sap vitality from your hair and leave it lifeless. You must have noticed how limp and dull it looked during your last bout with flu or grippe. Normally the vitality of your hair picks up as your strength and health return, but in cases of severe fever or a disease that shatters your entire system, you may suffer permanent baldness.

Stress and physical strain telescope your aging process and so can speed up the approach of white hair and baldness. Most men have just got to learn to take life a little more easy and learn to relax.

Your comb can kill. The comb you pass through your hair regularly throughout the day may actually be ruining it. Try this test. Run your thumbnail between the teeth at the point where they join the back of your comb. The surface should feel smooth. If the edges are sharp, they'll scrape your nail just as they scrape away at your hair every time you comb it. Recently I ran the test on the combs of a dozen or so men at a party. Five failed. Three of the most expensive-looking ones were the worst offenders. As with so many grooming aids, cost is no guarantee of quality. By the way, the women's combs were not much better.

Wet hair is in its most elastic state, so comb it gently. If you have long hair, start combing at the ends and work up, bit by bit, to the scalp. This will eliminate most of the tangles and consequent tugging which can damage hair.

Now that you know the basics of keeping your hair healthy and attractive-looking, your next step is to put it into the style that flatters you most.

STYLE YOUR HAIR TO MAKE MORE OF YOURSELF

The style in which men wear their hair tells a lot about them—swinger or square, director or clerk, good taste or bad. Not so long ago men had their hair cut only to get rid of it. Now the smart ones cut it to build an image, one that flatters the hell out of themselves. How about you? What does your hairstyle tell those in your firm or complete strangers at cocktail parties about you? Couldn't it say something better?

WHAT'S THE RIGHT STYLE FOR YOU?

The best hairstyle for you looks natural and blends unnoticeably with the rest of your physical and psychological makeup. Yet, in a subtle way, it should make you look more handsome than you are.

Your style should keep up with the current fashion, but it would be madness to adopt a new cut just to look trendy if it looks ridiculous on you. Sadly many men do this. Think of all those television commentators and late night show personalities who made the mistake of growing long hair regardless of their age in an attempt to appear "with it." (I hope their jobs weren't that insecure.) Also, it's foolish to stick to an outmoded style that makes you look outmoded, too. Be sensible. Compromise between what fits the trends and what flatters you most.

Enough theory; let's get practical. Thirty minutes in a barber chair may do more for you than a trip to an Austrian rejuvenation clinic. Look at your hair in relation to the following factors to see how you can turn it into a more flattering asset.

It improves your facial features

Your style should balance and soften overdominant features of your face. If you've got protruding ears, minimize them by growing your hair fuller at the sides to fill in the space and partially cover them. Lower a too high forehead by dipping your hair across it.

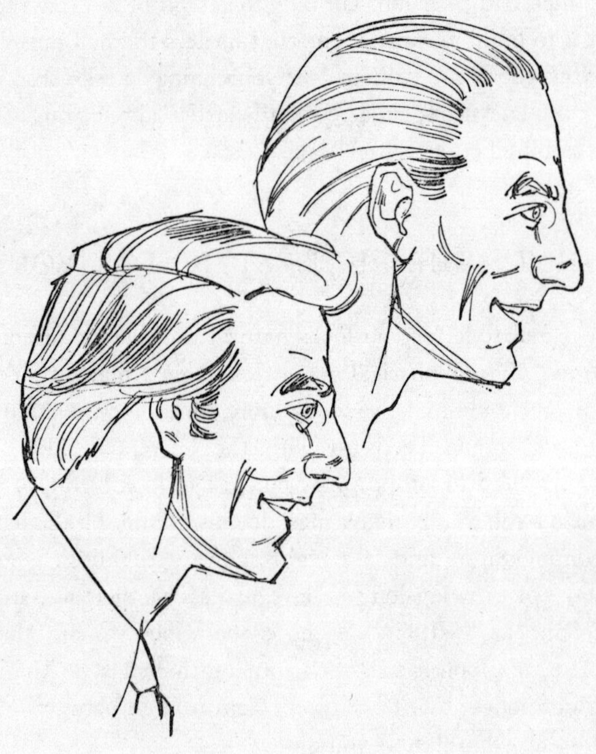

You can balance and make a large nose a flattering personality feature by combing your hair forward before letting it fall back in an abbreviated Elvis Presley style. Never comb your hair straight back from your forehead in this situation or you'll focus all attention on your nose. Some scars or birth marks may be hidden by your hair. The variations are unlimited, so experiment.

It flatters your body and build

The height and build of your body, if extreme in any way, should also be considered. For example, very heavy builds take more balancing hair on the head than slight ones; tall men more than short. But don't go to the lengths of those very short women who try to measure up to their boyfriends with beehive hairdos that add a good foot to the top of their heads. What good is all that distortion when their noses still bump their lovers' navels? I'd rather have a well-proportioned doll.

It builds a success image

Match your hairstyle to your existing image if that image works well for you. If not, style it to fit more closely the image of the typical, successful man in your professional or social environment. A haircut can turn an athlete into an executive or a liberal into a conservative, but remember, an image also combines your physical appearance, personality, and mode of dress. A freaked-out hairstyle fits well in trendy gear, but looks a bit out of place on top of a pin-striped suit in the executive suite. You can't be all things to all people, so make up your mind.

It knocks years off your age

As a general rule, most men under thirty can wear their hair in almost any style they want and look good. After thirty, the rules change. Take a long look at yourself. Does your current hairstyle really suit you? If it doesn't, invariably the answer will be that your hair is too long.

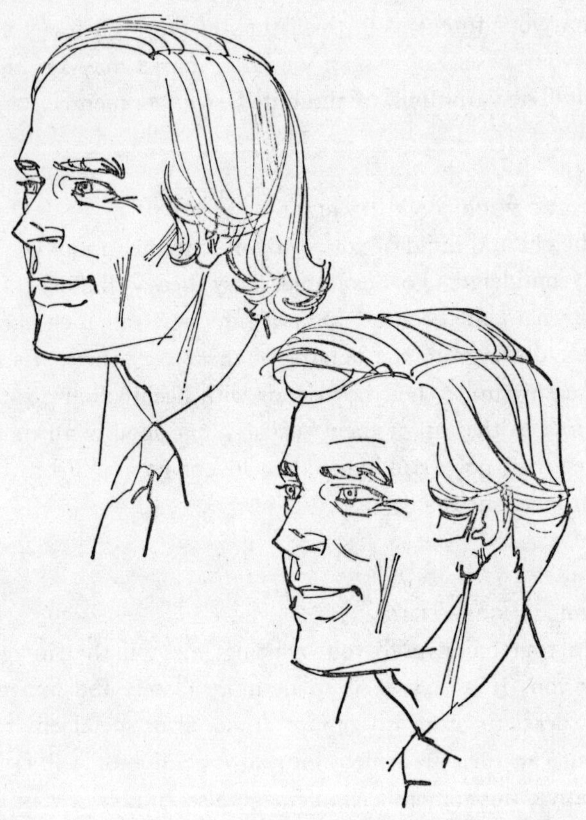

Shorter hair usually flatters and makes older faces look younger than long hair, no matter what the fashion. But don't go overboard. The Joe College crew cut would look pretty silly on Methuselah.

IT SUITS THE QUALITY OF YOUR HAIR

Finally, take into account the inherited quality of your hair—its shape, texture, and growth pattern—when styling it. Don't try to force your hair into a style it's physically incapable of holding. Three distinct hair shapes are features of racial origin:

Oriental hair is typically round in cross section and so behaves like a column trying to remain straight. It seems to have a mind of its own and resists being combed close to the head or put into more complicated styles.

Caucasian hair is usually wavy by nature, and its kidney-shaped cross section allows it to bend and fall over easily. Its curliness depends on the degree to which the follicles through which the hair grows are curved in your scalp. Caucasian hair is the easiest to manipulate.

Negroid hair generally has a very flat oval shape and a highly curved follicle which combine to make it extremely curly (kinky) and difficult to manage. It grows in its own natural style.

Interracial mixing has caused many variations of these three basic hair shapes.

Fine-textured hair doesn't have the body needed for many styles; it certainly won't go into an Afro. Adapt your visual ideas to fit your hair type and don't demand the impossible or you'll have to keep a comb in your hand every minute of the day.

Select your barber carefully

In his poem "The Rape of the Lock" Alexander Pope realized the disaster one can suffer at the hands of an unskilled barber. How good is yours? Many men can cut hair; the trick is to do more. Because of the increased demands by men for hair "styling," good barbers (or hairdressers) now use many of the techniques proved successful in working with women's hair. The excessive razor thinning so popular with men in the 1950s is out and has been replaced by scissors cutting, which gives the barber much greater control over your hair. He can better measure and cut it so each hair falls more naturally into place. Thus the over-all shape of your style becomes easier for you to maintain despite growth and repeated washing.

If used carefully by an expert, a razor may be all right, but risky. The problem lies with a razor in the hands of a barber who wields it like a sculptor to quick-thin your hair and carve it into a smooth-tapered shape that looks fine initially but seldom lasts that way very long. Every actor I know on both sides of the Atlantic insists on scissors cutting to keep his hair looking better for long periods of time, particularly when on tour. If you haven't already had a scissors cut, try one. You should be very happy with the difference.

Finally, the hairline at the nape of your neck should be soft, not a sharp, cleary defined line. If you keep your hair short, the barber should create a graduation in hair length from your clean-shaven neck up. Longer hairstyles should be kept fuller and softer at the back. Under no circumstances should your barber cut a straight line across the nape of your neck.

HOW TO CONTROL UNMANAGEABLE HAIR

Do you control your hair, or does it control you? Does it float about after washing, bristle with static electricity, or behave like barbed wire? Do you always run a comb quickly through it before going into your next meeting? You shouldn't have these problems if you follow part or all of the following grooming regimen.

FIRST COMES PROPER CUTTING AND CLEANING:

As we discussed earlier, the basis for good control lies in having your hair cut well and styled to suit its particular shape, texture, and pattern of growth. You must also keep it clean with regular shampooing so it doesn't get oily and go limp.

NEXT, "SET" YOUR HAIR

You may not realize it, but every time you wash, comb, and dry your hair, you're giving it a "set" similar to those that women get in their salons. If your hair gives you trouble, this is one of the easiest and most effective ways to tame it.

After shampooing, comb your damp hair into the style you want and cover it with a hairnet to keep it in place. (The tighter the net, the closer your hair will lie to the scalp.) Let it dry naturally, or speed up the process with an electric hair dryer. (Many inexpensive dryers are now made for men, or borrow your wife's.) When you remove the net, your hair will probably look plastered down, but should be well set into position unless you have very fine hair. Run a comb slowly through it to lift the hair up from your scalp and loosen it into a more natural look. Make any minor alterations by wetting parts of your hair with the comb and rearranging them.

You can use a water set to put temporary waves in your hair. Roll your damp hair tightly around a comb and dry it. Make sure you don't injure the hair with too much heat from your dryer. When you remove the comb, your hair should stay in a loose wave. An electric comb/dryer combination makes this type of styling very easy.

There's nothing mysterious about setting your hair—it's a natural phenomenon. The tiny fibers in your hair are linked together by bonds in much the same way the sides of a ladder are linked by rungs. Water affects some of them (the hydrogen bonds), and certain chemicals affect the others (chemical bonds). When you wash your hair, moisture penetrates it and breaks the hydrogen bonds apart. As your hair dries, the bonds relink in new pairs depending upon the bend you've put in it. The new bonds hold your hair in the same position that it dried, and will continue to hold it from within until moisture once again breaks the bonds.

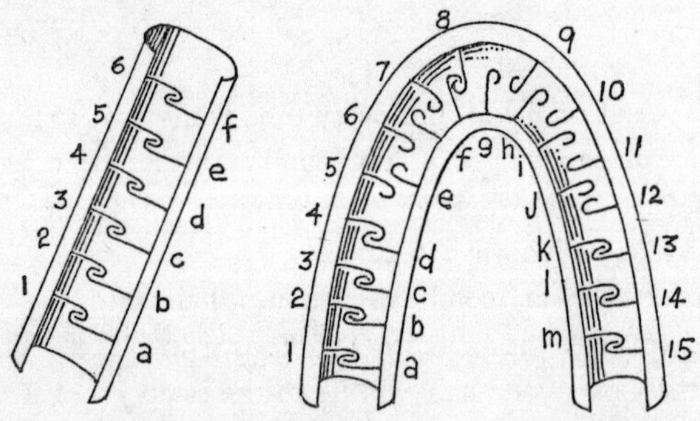

The chemical bonds are stronger than the hydrogen bonds and can only be broken by chemical action. Permanent waving lotions contain the chemicals to break these bonds. After the lotion has done its work and the hair has been arranged in the right style, a neutralizer refixes the bonds in new pairs. The new bonds are so strong, they can hold a tight wave through many shampoos and may last until the permanent grows out with the hair. That's why men use permanents to straighten very curly hair or to put body and curl into straight hair. Most of the more sophisticated men's hairdressers now offer you this service.

Apply a dressing to restore hair's natural sheen

After drying, use the dressing best suited to your hair's condition and texture. If you have **dry to normal hair,** use an oil dressing to replace some of the natural oil removed from your hair during shampooing. It will restore your hair's natural sheen, eliminate static electricity, and give it slightly more body to help hold it in place. Oil dressings must be used very sparingly to avoid a greasy look—a little goes a long, long way. One brand quite rightly advertised that "a little dab will do you."

Those of you with **normal to oily hair** should use a resin dressing. These brands are emulsions of resin in alcohol and water or thicker substances depending on the viscosity of their form. They coat your hair with a fine film of resin which hardens to hold it in place. This film also gets rid of static electricity, but may have the disadvantage of making your hair feel a bit stiff.

Use a hair spray for real problem hair

When used properly, and in the right strength for your particular control problem, resin sprays effectively hold your hair for long periods in situations of high activity. Once combed in place, the sprays stick your individual hairs together to form a sort of mat. Read the directions carefully because, although the packaging looks similar, the contents differ widely. The more resin a spray contains, the more its holding power. The stronger formulations are useful if you want to hold thinning hair over bald patches or have very fine textured hair.

Aerosol spray dressings have become popular with men because they're clean and easy to use. Unfortunately, they can leave your hair looking dull if overused, and, if not washed out, tend to flake off in a form of synthetic dandruff. Shampoo your hair frequently to eliminate these problems.

Of course, learning how to control your hair is essential for those of you who have hair to control, but what about your less fortunate contemporaries who are on their way to being bald? This takes us into a completely different problem area.

HAIR RECESSION AND BALDNESS

Some hair recession and thinning is common to us all as we age. But at what point does one suddenly realize that normal recession has turned into a full-scale route? One in every five Caucasian men will go bald. Will you be one of them?

THE CAUSES OF BALDNESS

Before you can understand baldness and how best to treat it, you've got to know how your hair grows and replaces itself. **Papillae** are the essential organs from which your hair grows. Like tiny factories, they lie deep in your scalp where blood vessels supply them with all the materials they need to manufacture hair. The strength and character of your hair depends on the inherited productivity of your papillae and the nourishment they get from your blood. No amount of "fertilizer" you pour over your head will have any affect on them.

Now comes the problem. When through inherited programming or other causes your papillae can't go on producing strong, healthy hair, they start turning out more delicate and degenerate hair. Finally they may appear to have stopped work all together, but this isn't so. Look carefully and you'll see most bald men's scalps still show a fuzz of fine hair growing there.

WHAT ABOUT THE HAIR IN YOUR SINK EVERY MORNING?

It's not as serious as you think. Your hair constantly sheds and replaces itself. The average growth cycle of hair runs about three years, although it can be as long as six. At the end of its cycle, each hair detaches itself from its papilla and moves up the follicle until it falls out. The papilla remains at rest for a while and then starts synthesizing material for a new hair. Hair grows about six inches a year. The longest hair ever recorded belonged to Swami Pandarasannadi, head of the Theravada Thurai Monastery in India. It was twenty-six feet long. (Thank Buddha there was no Mrs. Pandarasannadi!)

Most men have about 120 square inches of scalp, and about 1,000 hairs to each square inch. Thus you may have up to 120,000 hairs on top of your head. So don't worry too much when you see some in your comb and sink every day. You can afford to lose quite a few—as long as they're being replaced.

Heredity can cause baldness

By far the most common cause of baldness is heredity. If your family has a history of baldness, you're *likely* to inherit the tendency. (Some say it comes down through your mother's side of the family.) This problem occurs very gradually, usually starting in adolescence or early childhood, as the result of your body's reaction to the increased influence of male hormones. The reaction triggers off a change in the papillae so that instead of continuing to make strong hair, one after another starts turning out degenerate hair.

Preventing and treating hereditary baldness

The only sure way to prevent baldness is to choose a different set of parents, and the only known cure is castration (whatever else they may have lost, eunuchs from bald families don't lose their hair). Research is being done on antihormones to keep hair on top of your head while reducing beard growth to the point where you'd only have to shave once every few weeks. Not surprisingly, a breakthrough isn't anticipated for quite some time.

I hate to say it, but aside from the above, no way has yet been found to reverse or stop hereditary baldness no matter what the quacks claim. However, if caught early enough, it may be possible to forestall hair degeneration and baldness to some degree with proper treatment aimed at creating the healthiest possible environment for hair growth.

1. First, keep your hair and scalp as clean as possible. Stop excess oiliness, dryness, and scaling.

2. Protect it from too much sun, chemicals, rough massage, and other things that may harm it.

3. Keep physically healthy, stick to a good balanced diet, and mentally relax.

4. Have your hair and scalp checked periodically by dermatologists or qualified trichologists. *Warning:* A lot of unscrupulous operators run around advertising claims of hair restoration which usually involves rather expensive treatments. Their success stories probably come from patients who have suffered only temporary baldness from causes other than heredity. Don't be taken in. If diagnosed correctly by an expert, nonhereditary hair loss can usually be prevented, or at least contained; you're stuck with hereditary baldness.

Avoid the preventable causes of baldness

Your papillae will continue to live and produce hair until your body dies unless you kill them prematurely by a hard blow, deep scalp infection, a wound or burn. Severe damage to the follicles through which your hair grows can also cause permanent hair loss. A classmate of mine had a round bald patch right in the center of his hairline which was exactly the same size as the head of the hammer with which his younger brother clouted him years before.

Severe disease can put your papillae into a state of shock from which they may never recover. As mentioned before, prolonged illnesses which sap the strength of your general constitution can cause hair degeneration, and extreme diet deficiencies and certain scalp conditions may cause temporary or permanent baldness. Hair loss may also be brought on by scalp X rays and some medicines like several used to prevent blood clotting and a few drugs for the treatment of cancer. Your doctor will advise you on these hazards.

Stress can stimulate hair loss

As you go through this book, I hope you become more and more aware of the great damage stress and emotional strain inflict on all aspects of your health and looks. Simply worrying about baldness can actually speed up hair loss. Trichologists sometimes give placebo ointments and therapies to clients just to calm their fears and so help save their hair.

A common cause of bald patches is the nervous attack which you may be making on your hair this very moment without realizing it. This subconscious and nervous pulling of hair and rubbing your scalp creates irritation which leads to more rubbing and scratching and eventually to bald spots. Fortunately, you've only damaged your hair, not the papillae, so new hair will grow back as soon as you make a conscious effort to stop the attack.

HOW TO MAKE THE MOST OF BALDNESS

A lot of you are going to be bald and you've only got two ways to handle it: Either you make your peace and build baldness into a natural and distinguished part of your personality and appearance, or you fight back by covering it up. Whichever way you pick, you've got to do it well if you want to look attractive.

To make a success of the first approach, you must have sufficient confidence in yourself not to worry about what others think. During the early stages, style your hair to make its recession and thinning unnoticeable. As your hair loss becomes greater, gradually show it. A top international men's hairdresser (who also styles the hair of Princess Anne and other notables) told me, "It's death for men to cover up baldness if it can't be done well. They mustn't make others think they're embarrassed about it. People won't give your baldness a second glance unless you draw their attention to it by too obviously trying to hide it."

If you've got a completely bare crown, cut your side hair short so that it won't bush out to spoil the natural shape of your head. If long hair happens to be in fashion and it looks good on you, let your hair grow a bit longer at the nape of your neck. You might even go the whole way by shaving all of it off in the virile Yul Brynner style. Experiment. But for God's sake, don't stretch a few pathetic strands of hair across a shiny skull; you're not fooling anyone, and it's really ugly. Although baldness may add some years to the top of your head, you can take them back off by keeping your face and body in good trim.

The successful way to cover up hair loss

Through clever use of hair replacement and surgery, no one need ever know you don't have a full head of natural hair. Although a tricky and expensive route, it's a rewarding one. I know many men, some of them models and actors, who've had a fantastic success. I also know others who've made fools of themselves by trying to wear a pop singer's mop on top of a sixty-year-old face.

You may need one or all four of these hair replacement techniques before you're through: hair extension, toupees, wigs, and surgical transplants.

Hair extension, or weaving, effectively covers small bald patches. An expert knots hair, identical in texture and color to your own, into a light fabric base which he then anchors on your scalp by tying it to the natural hair surrounding the bald spot. When styled and cut together, the new hair extension should be completely indistinguishable from your own hair.

As the anchoring hairs grow, the base will rise with them, so you must return regularly to the fitter to have it pushed back down on your scalp. You can enter into strenuous activity without fear of dislodging the base, but I personally think the claims about being able to swim without problems have been exaggerated. To play safe, wear a swimming cap.

Use **toupees** (better called hairpieces) in increasing sizes as your hair loss increases. Like hair extension, hair is matched to your own and knotted into a fabric base, but the hairpiece is anchored directly to your scalp with adhesive. Because it doesn't rely on surrounding hair for security, you can bring a toupee forward to restore a youthful hairline. Comb your own hair over the toupee edges to conceal them. If you don't have any natural hair over your forehead, dip the toupee hair horizontally across your forehead or comb it forward and back to hide the front edge. Well-made toupees usually have short hair running along the front edge to help disguise it.

A hairpiece is a relatively delicate thing and can be dislodged, so don't wear it in physical-contact sports. Although a good toupee can be worn in swimming, it's best not to do it. Salt water and chlorinated water tend to affect the foundation and may loosen the hair knots. Also, they may change the color of the hair. Unless you want to impress someone, don't wear a toupee to bed because prolonged stress will warp it out of shape. A hairdresser should dry-clean a hairpiece regularly to remove scalp oils and dirt, and to keep it smelling fresh. The price of a good average-sized toupee (six inches by eight inches) runs between $275 and $400 depending upon the color of hair used. White hair costs the most, followed by pale blond. The darker colors are least expensive. Some imported Oriental hairpieces cost as little as $60—and look it.

Wigs cover your entire head like snug-fitting caps. You don't need adhesive to hold a good one in place. As with toupees, dip the hair across your forehead or brush it forward to disguise the front edge. If possible, blend it in with the hair around your ears and at the nape of your neck with a comb.

You've got to preserve your wig's snug fit as long as possible, so don't wear it in swimming, for contact sports, or in bed. It will need regular dry cleaning and styling, but usually not as often as a toupee. A good wig costs between $400 and $600 depending upon size and color.

TIPS ON BUYING HAIRPIECES

Don't be cheap. Unless you only want to wear it to a fancy dress ball for a giggle, don't waste your money on inferior hairpieces. They're obvious, or will be within a short time.

Check their color and texture. Your natural hair color contains a blend of several different colors, not just one. A good wig or hairpiece maker will use different shades to achieve the perfect match. As your hair grays, have your hairpiece changed to preserve the match.

If you have fine or coarse hair, make sure the hairpiece does, too. The same applies to hair shape. Cheap hairpieces often contain inexpensive Oriental hair, which may look quite different from your own and be difficult to control. Can you imagine the chaos if Negroid hair were mixed in as well? Few men's hairpieces contain synthetic hair because of its artificial, giveaway shine, and the colors aren't true. Some new synthetic fibers have recently been developed which come very close to natural-looking hair, but they don't yet stand up to close scrutiny.

Match hair density. The most common fault in toupees and wigs results from the demands of the men ordering them: too much hair. Don't go overboard and insist on lots of hair. As you age, your hair naturally thins a bit. Too dense a head of hair for your age won't look right and will set people to wondering. You don't want to encourage this type of speculation.

Hair transplants have become very popular because they offer a permanent solution to baldness. Several years ago a more youthful-looking Senator William Proxmire surprised his congressional colleagues with one. In this operation, tiny cores of scalp that contain papillae producing strong hair are cut from the nape of your neck and transplanted to the top of the head. The cores removed from the top replace those taken from the nape. A transplant is successful only when the blood vessels rearrange themselves to supply the new papillae with the materials they need for continued hair growth.

Transplants take time, can be painful, and aren't always successful. Also, they can't be performed on all people. Your scalp and papillae must be in the right condition. Your type and degree of baldness obviously represents another factor in determining what results you can expect from a transplant. If you have a bald spot of twenty square inches (not an uncommon size), you're missing about twenty thousand strands of hair. You can't expect to replace all twenty thousand from the nape of your neck; you'll need a lot just to give a thin, covered look. Transplants, therefore, appear most effective in adding to areas of existing thin hair and in combination with toupees, where transplanted hair can be used to hide the front edges of the foundation fabric.

Now that we've discussed the ways bald men can make themselves more attractive, what about those of you with graying hair?

MAKE GRAY HAIR AN ASSET

When talking about hair, most men seem to believe that only black is beautiful. Wrong—gray hair is extremely flattering, or can be if handled right. Every secretary in one of New York's biggest soap and detergent marketing companies would gladly have given more than her right arm to hop into bed with a rugged young executive whose prematurely silver-gray hair dazzled them. It used to drive his wife up the wall, not to mention the office efficiency experts.

HOW TO TREAT GRAY HAIR

Can natural hair color be restored?

First, let's get this obvious question out of the way. Gray hair is really hair with no color (white hair) mixed in with your regular hair to give an over-all gray effect. It creeps in when the programming of one papilla after another calls for it to stop putting pigment into the hair. Up to the age of thirty, the absence of color is considered "premature" and due to heredity. After that, colorless hair results from the natural aging process.

No way has yet been found to make the papillae produce pigment once they've stopped. However, the future holds some hope. As a side effect of cortisone treatments, some white-haired patients regained their natural hair color. Further research into the chemistry of pigment production may bring an end to gray hair, but right now the only way to restore your natural color is to dye your hair.

Style gray hair cleverly to make the most of it

When styling gray hair, remember two things: Except on obviously young men, gray hair ages you, and the longer your hair, the greater the visual impact of any white hair mixed in with the dark. Thus "salt and pepper" hair usually looks best when kept short. Because of a little gray, a lot of long-haired, middle-aged hippies look much older than their years.

If you've got a good bit of gray at your temples and want the distinguished, man-of-the-world look, don't cut it short. Instead comb it back over your ears to create an elegant line on each side of your head. Most women find it irresistible.

Silver your gray

Periodically, ask your barber to use a blue rinse or a semi-permanent dye to add a silver tint and highlights to your gray hair. This will keep it from going dull and yellowish. You can do it yourself, but go easy. You don't want to end up like one of those little old blue-haired ladies on Fifth Avenue or Bond Street, who also come in unusual shades of pink and purple.

Coloring gray hair

If you really hate the idea of going gray, start coloring it before it becomes too pronounced so no one will realize there's gray underneath. If your hair is already gray, color it gradually with several treatments over several weeks so you don't draw the attention of your friends and business associates to what you're doing. An international financier and ladies' man *extraordinaire* covered his gray hair this way and was a little disappointed that none of the women noticed what he considered his more youthful appearance. They must have been too distracted by another aspect of his physiology.

Several fine coloring products are sold for men, and their application is very easy. These products come in a limited range of colors. You might swallow your pride and use one of the semi-permanent coloring products "made for women." The basic formulations are the same as the men's products, but the wider color selection may enable you to get a better match with your natural hair color.

Gray hair "restorers," no matter what the advertised implication, are cover-up dyes, not papillae stimulators. They may look like clear liquids, but they contain a salt which oxidizes when exposed to air to coat white hair with a brown film. If you keep using them, the dye will eventually penetrate into your hair shafts for more or less permanent coloring.

If you choose to restore your original hair color with dyes and are in your forties or more, use a color one shade lighter than your original color. It will look much more natural and flatter your more mature skin tone. How's that for going one better than nature?

COLOR YOUR HAIR YOUNG

A brilliant New York architect, responsible for designing everything from hotels to sheikh's palaces, lunched with me at the beach several weeks ago. Although in his fifties, he could pass for forty. The reason? Aside from a good firm body, he had a youthful, attractive head of hair without a trace of gray. The only thing that suggested he had colored his hair was the gray on his chest.

Hair coloring represents about the closest thing you can get to the Fountain of Youth, but it can be tricky. Today men color their hair to disguise gray, lighten or darken nondescript hair, or streak it for the flattering, sun-bleached look of the athlete.

WHAT'S PERFECTLY COLORED HAIR?

Perfectly colored hair is discreet. It looks completely natural and fits your skin color. Nature created you as one harmonious unit, and radical hair-color changes seldom look right on a man. It can be summed up by adapting one of the most successful advertising campaigns for hair coloring preparations in recent years: "Does he, or doesn't he? Only his hairdresser knows for sure."

How to go about coloring your hair

Coloring gray hair to "restore" its natural, youthful look can be a relatively simple and successful operation if done gradually and with care. But approach the change of your hair color with thought and care. A botched job turns women off and lets you in for a lot of smug smiles. Discuss it with your barber or hairdresser and let him do it for you. Selecting the proper shade and right formulation for the texture and porosity of your hair calls for skill and experience which we men just don't have. Don't take chances. Decide upon the color you *think* you want to end with, and let your barber work toward it gradually in several sessions. You'll probably find that the color that best suits you falls very close to your own natural color. Minor changes of this sort can be very attractive and are relatively easy to maintain.

Above all, be honest with yourself. Not too long ago I chatted with a lesser television and theater personality who had strangely colored and dull hair. He has the reputation of being bitchy and hypercritical of everyone in the trade. He obviously forgot to turn his critical gaze in his own mirror.

Do-it-yourself

If you insist on going it alone, for God's sake be careful. Don't suddenly get the urge to take the plunge after a few martinis and swipe your girl friend's hair coloring.

1. Carefully choose the right preparation for the color and permanency you want. Various preparations can give you a temporary, minor color change or a more radical, permanent one. Try the temporary rinse as an experiment. Later use the semipermanent and permanent formulations as you become more skilled and see how color changes affect your appearance.

The color you get from a temporary rinse or a semipermanent brand combines the original color of your hair with the film of new color coating it. Permanent products can give a truer color change and also leave your hair a bit more lustrous than the flatter look from temporary preparations.

Temporary color products are usually rinsed into your hair after shampooing and left for a few minutes. They add highlights to your natural hair color, can change the tone of blond hair, and cover up or silver your gray hair. They're useful in reviving the color of hair faded by the action of sun and chlorine water, but have no lightening action. Temporary coloring lasts until you shampoo your hair again.

Semipermanent brands are shampooed or foamed into your hair and left up to forty-five minutes depending upon the intensity of color you desire. These preparations cover gray and add highlights to or deepen your natural hair color. They last through three to five shampoos.

Permanent products very in their application. They can lighten, darken, or change the natural color of your hair and cover up gray. The color change lasts until your hair grows out. To change dark hair into blond, you must first bleach out the original color and then replace it with a lighter one. As your hair grows, keeping its darker roots matching the lighter new color represents quite a chore. Also, bleached hair feels coarser to the touch. You may have experienced this when running your fingers through the hair of natural versus artificial blondes.

Streaking hair is simply bleaching the tips of some of the strands, not others. The theory may sound simple, but not the execution. Do-it-yourselfers court disaster. Be warned.

2. Before using the color preparation, test yourself for any allergic reaction to it by doing a skin-patch test, as explained on the package.

3. Read every last letter of the instructions and follow them exactly, particularly the timing directions in relation to the texture and porosity of your hair. The more porous your hair, the more dye it will take on.

4. Keep all formulations away from your eyes. Never apply them to your eyebrows.

5. Use conditioners more often to maintain good body and feel to your hair.

6. The best of luck!

An added thought—the psychology of hair color

Advertisers tell us that blondes have more fun than brunettes. There's more fact than fiction to this. Research shows women generally associate personality traits to various hair colors. They consider blondes to be less intelligent party girls, redheads as dynamic, fashion-setting vamps, and brunettes as intelligent and sophisticated. A woman's personality usually changes dramatically to fit more in line with the stereotyped image of her new hair color.

To my knowledge, little if any research in this area has been conducted on men. By changing your hair color, you strike out in psychologically virgin territory. Don't be surprised if you see a seventy-year-old gentleman with newly streaked hair riding a surfboard in Malibu!

IMPROVE YOUR LOOKS BY REMOVING HAIR

Being attractive and well groomed depends not only on taking care of the hair on top of your head, but the hair all over the rest of your body. In many cases, like shaving your beard, this means getting rid of it. The average man doesn't realize the importance of removing unwanted hair, so you have a competitive edge.

Next time you're in a meeting, look at the men around the table. How many have straggly eyebrows and hair sticking out of their noses? As you age, the growth and coarseness of superfluous hair increases everywhere on your body except your scalp, where you want it most. Just because nature gives you this added bonus doesn't mean you have to keep it. Well-turned-out men don't. They know the best way to groom their eyebrows, get rid of stray hairs on or in their noses, and how to remove hair permanently from their shoulders and back. It improves their sex appeal and looks; why not yours?

GROOM YOUR EYEBROWS TO LIGHTEN YOUR FACE

Eyebrows often dominate your appearance and expression. I don't advocate radically altering or reshaping them, just keeping them tidy. Usually a dozen or so hairs grow on the bridge of your nose between the eyebrows. They add nothing to the shape and line of your brows; instead they give you a shaggy and neglected look. Get rid of them.

Sometimes eyebrows grow straight across the nose, creating a scowling, thunderous expression. Unless this image suits you and you enjoy frightening little children, as an acquaintance of mine does, consider removing the bridging hair. It can lighten your face and may give you a more open and youthful expression. Before taking the step, however, visualize the difference by sticking a piece of skin-colored tape over the unwanted hair. If you decide to go ahead, remove the hair gradually, making sure not to create too abrupt and artificial a line between your brows and the skin separating them. Thin the hair at the edges a bit so it will look as if your brows just petered out naturally.

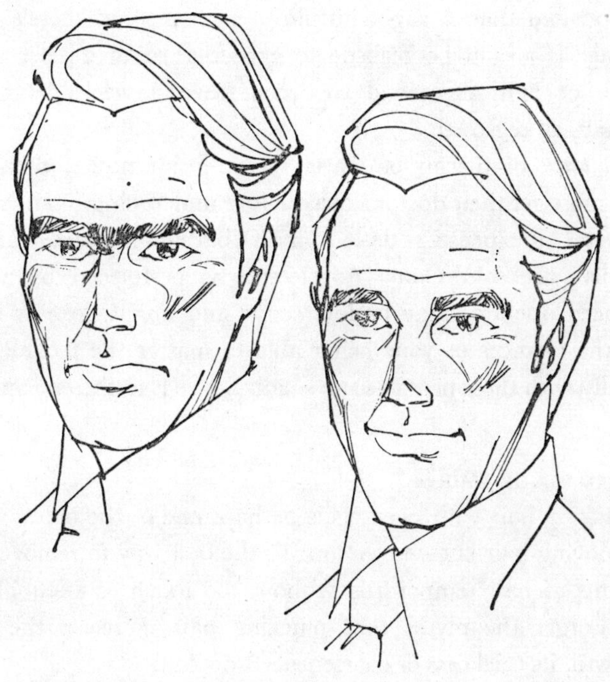

Your goal in removing hair is to do it so others won't know it was ever there. Its absence shouldn't appear unnatural or be missed, and no stubble should draw attention to your efforts. Shaving is a poor method for removing hair other than your beard because it leaves a stubble visible within a day or two at the most. Plucking or diathermy are your best bets for removing hair on your face and body.

Electrolysis

Diathermy is the newer, faster, and most popular electrolysis technique. It offers you a reasonable assurance of permanent hair removal. The electrologist inserts a fine wire needle into your follicles to kill the papillae with electric current. Done properly, you'll feel no more than a slight burning sensation, and there's no skin scarring. It would be realistic to expect a 10 to 25 per cent regrowth of hair. A second treatment several weeks later should eliminate all regrowth.

Don't use diathermy on warts, moles, inside nose and ears. Diabetics must get their doctor's okay before undergoing treatments.

Several inexpensive do-it-yourself battery-operated diathermy "pencils" are sold today. As electrolysis performed by an inexperienced operator may be ineffective and might possibly damage skin, the chances of your being able to master the technique successfully with these pencils seem small. Leave it to the experts.

How to pluck hair

Plucking hair with tweezers is perhaps one of the oldest methods of removing hair known to man. It's the best way to remove limited amounts of hair temporarily without too much of a stubble problem. Forget the myths that plucking hair increases the rate of regrowth, its thickness or coarseness. It doesn't.

You can pluck hair more easily from skin softened and relaxed with hot, wet towels or a shower or bath. After removing hair this way, it's a good idea to splash the area with a little alcohol. An astringent after-shave lotion or cologne should do the job.

REMOVE NOSE HAIR

Pluck or remove by diathermy (don't shave) the few hairs that may grow on top of your nose. They're not only unattractive, but age you. Have you seen young men with them? Seldom, if ever.

When hair growing within your nose becomes so long that it sticks out, carefully trim it back with a pair of round-tipped scissors. Don't pull it out because of the chance of infection. Often good barbers will automatically trim your nose hair without thinking to ask. If they consider it a common, good grooming practice, shouldn't you?

DON'T FORGET YOUR EARS

As with your nose, carefully trim any hair growing out of or on your ears. Use round-tipped scissors to avoid possible damage to your skin and don't put them far into your ear. I'd rather have fuzzy ears than deaf ones.

TIDY UP YOUR BODY HAIR

Pluck or use diathermy to remove those stray hairs growing on your shoulders or back. If you want to get rid of large areas of hair completely, do it permanently. Put yourself in the hands of a good electrologist who will do the job over a period of months so the process of hair removal will be gradual and not obvious to others. (Special rates can usually be obtained on a course of treatments.) Don't use a razor or depilatory or you'll land yourself with a mammoth stubble problem; your wife can vouch for this from her leg experience.

Sometimes hair under the arms, around the nipples, on the chest, or elsewhere on your body grows too long and makes you look more shaggy than virile. Simply trim or thin it a bit from time to time with round-tipped scissors and a comb. It takes little skill and less effort. Just don't go so far that you look like a clipped chicken rather than someone with a normally hairy body. You'll soon get the hang of it and cut a much snappier and more attractive figure on the beach or while having morning coffee in bed.

I'll end this section with your most common hair removal problem—your beard.

HOW TO GET A GOOD, CLOSE SHAVE

First, choose your weapon

Both safety razors and electric razors give you a good shave when properly used, so there's no point in my trying to switch you from one to the other. Use the one that is most comfortable. Blades usually give you a closer shave, but electric razors are faster and more convenient to use. Anyway, as most men have to shave twice a day if they want a really smooth face for both morning and evening activities, I see little practical difference between the two methods. Bear in mind only one point of difference which has importance in taking care of your skin: wet shaving dries your skin more than electric and should generally be followed by the use of a moisturizer.

Forget the shaving myths. Neither electric nor safety razors change the rate of your hair growth, its quality, or its thickness. Your beard gets coarser over the years because of age, not your razor. If either method did increase hair growth and texture, you could be sure every balding man in America would be shaving his scalp regularly.

Next, use a magnifying mirror

You can remove only what you can see. A magnifying shaving mirror will help you get a much closer shave, particularly on the tip of your chin and under it.

Prepare your whiskers

You stand up your whiskers for easier and closer shaves either by surrounding them with an excess of moisture or by an absence of moisture.

Wet shave preparation:
After washing or rinsing your face in warm water apply your shaving cream. Aerosol lather preparations have become popular purely because of their convenient form. They offer no additional benefits to your face or shaving performance over more traditional forms.
Like most shaving creams, aerosols usually contain an emulsion of water and various oils, plus perfume. When released from the can, the expanding propellent becomes trapped by the surrounding oil and water emulsion to form the tiny bubbles of the lather.
The oil lubricates your skin and the cream stands up your whiskers by holding water against them. The cream also forms an emulsion with your

Electric shave preparation:
Your skin may often be dry enough so your whiskers stand up and your razor moves smoothly over your skin without the need for a preshave preparation. At other times, perspiration or moisture from a steamy bathroom may soften your whiskers and inhibit razor movement so you get a spotty and far from close shave.
In these cases, apply a preshave lotion. It usually contains alcohol to get rid of perspiration and dry and stiffen your whiskers, and a little oil to lubricate your skin so the razor will move over it easily without biting in.

The cutting surface:
The cutting blades or head of your electric razor should be kept clean and sharp. Remove

natural skin oils and dirt, holding them in suspension until scraped away by your razor.

The razor blade:
As your blade sharpness is important to a comfortable and close shave, never dull it by wiping it with a towel or tissue. Just rinse under hot water.
Change your blade whenever it starts to tug at, rather than slice through, your whiskers.

After shaving:
Some manufacturers suggest you rub any cream left on your face into your skin to replace some of the natural oils your blade has scraped away. Because of the wide range of preparations (and their different additives) on the market, I recommend against this general practice.
Rinse your face thoroughly with warm water to remove any leftover cream. Apply an after-shave lotion or cologne to cotton and wipe your face. These astringent preparations (basically alcohol, water, and perfume) wake up your skin and clean away excess oil.
Splash your face twelve times with cold water and towel almost dry.

skin oil and hair from them regularly and follow the manufacturer's instructions concerning sharpening. Remember that the cutting surfaces may not have the same effective life-span as the motor, so be prepared to replace them if they become dull or worn.

After shaving:
Clean your face. Apply an astringent after-shave lotion or cologne to cotton and wipe your face to remove excess oil. Refer to the next chapter for the best care for your particular type of skin.
Rinse your face twelve times in cold water and towel almost dry. Gently rub a moisturizing cream, oil, or lotion into your skin (unless it's naturally oily) to help it retain moisture. Some after-shaving lotions now contain a little oil for moisturizing purposes and supposedly enable you to tone and moisturize your skin at the same time. I personally prefer separating the two steps with the cold water rinse.

Apply a moisturizing cream, oil, or lotion to your skin (unless it's naturally oily) to help it retain moisture. Refer to the next chapter for the best care for your skin type.

CHAPTER 3

Skin: How to Put Your Best Face Forward

In work, the successful man puts his best face forward as well as his best foot. Therefore it's important for you to have a really good complexion and keep it looking youthful, fresh, and attractive.

Men from all walks of life—celebrities down to struggling young businessmen—are now improving their skin with the care it has always needed. Those with really attractive wives want to keep up by looking just as handsome as their wives do beautiful. With a little prodding from their women, men now make up a third of the clientele in some of Los Angeles' best facial salons.

But if you think improving your skin means sitting for hours in a salon and slapping on layers of expensive, highly scented day and night creams, lotions, and masks, you're wrong. The skin care regimen in this book isn't founded on psychological dream advertisements, but on facts. It cuts through the cosmetic nonsense and goes right to the basics of what your skin really needs. It's simple and easy to follow—and it works. Give it only thirty days and see if you aren't happier with the results.

PERFECT SKIN

What are you aiming for? Perfect skin is basically young, unblemished skin. It looks smooth and feels soft. It's neither greasy nor dry. The pores have not become enlarged to spoil its fine texture. It has muscle tone, firmness, and elasticity and so is supple and free from wrinkles.

Your skin surface and pores should be free of stale oil, dirt, and blackheads and have a healthy pink color radiating from within. Finally, it shouldn't be inflamed or marred with pimples, herpes, or the many other common skin afflictions which can attack it.

The differences between the quality and texture of men's skins result from four basic factors: heredity, diet, general health, and the care they take of their skin. One man may start off life with a better-looking skin than another but, through neglect, end up with a far worse one.

THE BASICS OF GOOD SKIN CARE

Good skin care does two things. It helps offset the effects of the natural aging process on your skin, and it protects your skin from environmental conditions and other enemies that deteriorate it.

How to offset the effects of age

Your skin is divided into two distinct layers differing entirely in their structure: the outer layer, the epidermis, and the underlying layer, the dermis.

The epidermis, sometimes called your scarf skin, consists of cells clinging tightly together to form a resistant tissue which defends your body against its environment. The protective outer cells of the epidermis are tough and mostly dead. They rub off or are shed by your body only to be replaced with new cells growing up from the inner layer of the epidermis. This layer contains rich supplies of blood vessels which form a nourishing environment for cell growth. On an average, you shed about one gram in weight of skin cells every day. It's this rapid cell replacement that keeps your skin looking fresh and youthful and enables worn and injured skin to renew itself.

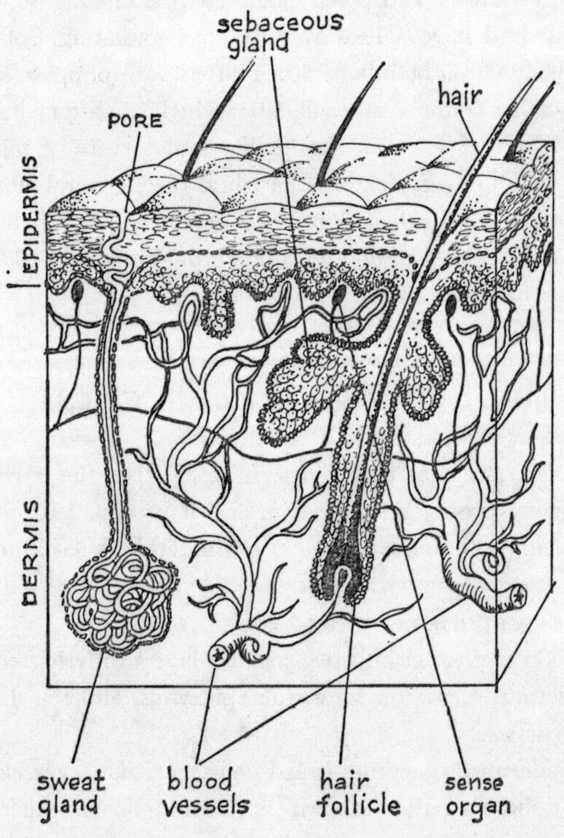

The dermis makes up most of your skin's thickness. It contains a dense network of connective fibers mixed with elastic fibers (formed from collagen, the basic intercellular material) which give your skin its pliability while keeping it firm and taut. The dermis also contains sensory nerves and the blood vessels which supply nourishment to your skin. In addition, it holds vast numbers of oil and sweat glands which affect the condition of your skin and so are vital to its health and good looks.

Your skin passes through several stages as you mature. Its gradual degeneration can be slowed with the right care, but not reversed.

As a youth, you share many characteristics with girls: hair in the same places, similar skin texture, and dry skin. When puberty approaches, the increased influence of the male hormones in your body stimulates the growth of facial and body hair and increases the oiliness of your skin. It's at this time that your acne or pimple problems start. Young men must take especially good care of their skin during this period to reduce the risk of scars which may last a lifetime. (See the section on dermabrasion, page 87.)

At around the age of twenty (this differs with each person) the body gradually reduces its production of oil, and from that time on, your skin becomes less oily and progressively drier. You should compensate for some of this oil reduction to keep your skin from losing too much internal moisture and becoming overly dry.

With age, cell replacement slows, causing a deterioration of your epidermis which becomes flaky and scaly. This, coupled with increasing dryness, results in a poor skin surface filled with tiny cracks and crevices in which bacteria happily multiply and impurities collect to irritate it. As its ability to renew itself decreases, you must take greater care to protect your skin from harsh environments and clean it more gently.

Wrinkles start making their appearance when the elastic collagen fibers in the dermis which keep the skin taut and flexible begin to degenerate. There's little you can do to compensate for this process. Other than cosmetic surgery, using a moisturizer to help your skin remain plump is the best long-term way to stretch out and minimize tiny wrinkles.

Protect your skin from its enemies

Every day you expose your complexion to things that can harm it and speed its degeneration. Your common sense and a little caution will help keep it looking younger.

As a child the skin of your face and body looked the same, but as you matured and your face bore the brunt of the effects of sun, wind, and water, the difference between the two became obvious. Your facial skin developed a coarser texture, particularly evident among farmers and sailors with whom we associate the rugged weather-beaten look. Fortunately, the glands in your facial skin and scalp produce more oil than those of the rest of your body, so these exposed areas get additional protection against hostile environments. The hotter the weather, the more oil produced to protect your skin from the dehydrating effects of the sun and perspiration. It's as if nature were applying a moisturizer to the skin. You should give nature a hand by protecting your skin as much as possible from extreme, hostile environments.

Beware of the sun. We generally consider tanned skin to be healthy. It is not. Tanned skin is damaged skin. Chronic overexposure to sun seriously degenerates your skin. (See the following chapter.)

Avoid physical damage to your skin. Obviously any external action, friction, or extremes of temperature that wound, callous, blister, burn, or freeze your skin will harm it. Wear the proper protective clothing whenever possible.

Chemical reactions and allergies can make your skin most unattractive and uncomfortable. No manufactured product exists to which someone, somewhere in the world, isn't allergic. Chemical substances may irritate and inflame your skin as can foods and other natural products to which you are oversensitive. Cases have been reported of husbands developing allergic skin reactions to their wives—rather interesting grounds for divorce. Although reputable manufacturers conduct extensive tests on all products that will come in contact with your skin, sooner or later you're likely to run into one that will bring you out in a rash or bumps. At the first sign of discomfort, trace the offending product and get rid of it.

Soap, on the whole, causes very little skin trouble if not overused to the point of removing too much of your skin's natural oils. A few people may develop an allergy to the perfume or some other ingredient in a particular brand of soap, but by switching to another or using a special additive-free soap, they overcome this problem.

Detergents, on the other hand, are not usually designed for use on the skin because of their great effectiveness in dissolving and removing oil. If you're washing dishes, clothing, or anything else with a detergent or one of the biological washing powders containing enzymes which split protein, make sure you rinse your hands thoroughly.

Water hardness, in itself, has little or no effect on your skin. Contrary to what many people think, hard water doesn't "clog" your pores. It does, however, diminish the ability of soap to clean and combines with soap to leave a thin film over your skin. By adding softeners to your bath water, you'll increase the cleaning efficiency of soap and reduce the film on your skin.

Diet: The quality of your skin relies upon a diet sufficient to supply all the needs of your body; heredity, which controls to some extent how your body utilizes that diet; and general good health, which enables all your organs to function effectively to make proper use of the food. In health, at least 95 per cent of all men living in the affluent Western societies have diets sufficiently varied to supply all their needs for healthy skin. Good skin needs vitamins A and B_1, found in animal foods (meat, fish, milk, and eggs), vegetables, and fruit. A good varied diet includes these things, so don't worry unless you decide to go on some wild crash diet. Then check with your doctor.

HOW TO IMPROVE YOUR COMPLEXION AND KEEP IT LOOKING YOUNGER

1. FIRST, DETERMINE YOUR SKIN TYPE

You've got to know your skin type so you can select the products and regimen best suited to your skin's needs. Your skin may be oily, normal, or dry depending upon the activity of its sebaceous glands. These oil glands take raw materials from the surrounding blood vessels and produce a fatty substance (called sebum) which they secrete into your hair follicles and through ducts opening directly onto the surface of your skin. The sebum lubricates your hair and gives pliability to your skin surface. This coating of oil helps your skin retain the moisture it needs to stay plump and fight wrinkles.

Your face probably combines two types of skin, one over the cheeks and the other in a center panel including the center of your forehead, your nose and the skin immediately on each side, and your chin. Like many men, you may have dry cheeks and an oily or nor-

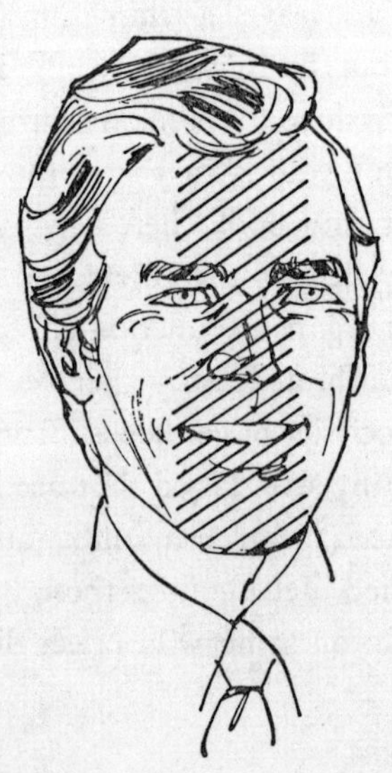

mal center panel. Analyze your facial and body skin using the following guidelines. Do it in the morning before bathing or shaving when your skin is in its natural state.

Oily skin usually has a coarse, often open-pored appearance, caused by the overactivity of the sebaceous glands clogging and stretching its pores. The skin has a sallow color and develops blackheads and spots easily. Although prevalent among teen-agers, this condition by no means disappears at the magic age of twenty-one, and may dog you for life. Oily-skinned men may have difficulty looking healthy because they lack the high coloring of those with dry or normal skin. Its main advantage is that it stands up well to age and doesn't wrinkle easily. Proper care calls for removing excess oil and keeping the skin clean and the pores unclogged.

Dry skin is common to young boys and older men and generally feels taut, as if it were being drawn tightly across your skull. Rarely troubled by acne and spots, it has small pores, which help make a good complexion, but sometimes it looks a bit scaly and rough. Unfortunately, dry skin doesn't stand up well and wrinkles easily with age. This skin type is characterized by tiny feather veins, especially on the cheeks, and high coloring. You should balance it through proper cleaning and use moisturizers to bring it nearer to the normal skin type.

Normal skin: We'd all like to be born with the normal skin type. You can identify it because it won't fall into the other two categories. It has none of the extreme advantages or disadvantages of the other types; not unduly troubled with spots and excessive oiliness, nor does it feel taut. Aim your care at maintaining your skin in this condition as long as possible.

2. Next, clean your skin to suit its condition

You clean your skin for three reasons: to remove dirt and grease accumulated during the day and get rid of alien or toxic substances which might irritate it. You also want to remove excess sebum and unplug your pores to help stop blackheads, pimples, and spots.

How clean is clean? Cleanliness may be next to godliness, but it can be overdone. Dermatologists generally consider healthy skin properly cleaned when a tissue rubbed over the face (or body) picks up no grease or dirt marks. Young people can seldom overdo cleaning their skin. Old people can. As skin ages and produces less oil and perspiration, it doesn't need as frequent cleaning. Overcleaning, particularly with soap and water, can remove too much natural oil and cause dryness and irritation.

The best ways to clean normal to oily skin

Normal to oily skin can be effectively cleaned in many ways. From the following alternatives, select the method which best suits your skin, makes it feel soft and smooth without drying it:

Soap and water does a good job on oily and on normal skin if not overused. Soap removes oil and dirt from your skin by both physical and chemical action. The physical action of rubbing soap and water over your face and body does most of the job.

Super-fatted soaps have greater than normal fatty acid content and therefore make more stable and luxurious lather on your skin. Use this type of soap in hard water areas where regular soaps don't lather well.

Deodorant soaps, in addition to their cleaning properties, contain bacteriostat ingredients which leave a very fine film on your skin to inhibit the growth of odor-causing bacteria.

Special medicated soaps come in liquid and solid form. Boys and men with excessively oily problem skin should use these to help during adolescence when acne trouble strikes in full force, and may need them long after that. Your doctor or pharmacist can recommend the best one for your particular skin problem.

Detergent bars are synthetic soap and have greater ability to dissolve and remove grease than soap. Because of this property, detergent bars can rob your skin of too much natural oil and dry it. Use them only on excessively oily skin.

Bath versus shower: You can clean your skin more effectively by bathing in a tub than taking a shower because your entire body comes into contact with the physical and chemical action of soap and warm water for a longer time. A shower, on the other hand, is less drying and so more advantageous for those with dry body skin. A slight added bonus: You'll keep your summer tan longer if you take showers.

Men's colognes and most after-shave lotions are astringents. As such, they can effectively remove natural skin oil, cleansing cream, and traces of shaving cream from your face. Thus astringents are a useful tool in cleaning oily skin, but if you have dry or normal skin, always follow astringents with a moisturizer to replace some of the lost natural oil.

When used for cleaning, apply an astringent to cotton and gently wipe your face. Repeat this action until the cotton no longer picks up any trace of oil or dirt. Astringents usually contain a mixture of water, alcohol, and perfume. Some have minor amounts of various additives like alum, menthol, and glycerin to further tighten and cool your skin and to make it feel smooth.

Shaving creams clean your skin as well as prepare your beard for the razor. They usually combine the various oils found in soaps with water, perfume, and additives like menthol. Shaving cream, like soaps and cleansing creams, form an emulsion with the dirt and oil on your skin which your razor physically scrapes away.

Wet shaving, therefore, removes natural oil which can benefit men with oily skin. Conversely, it has an adverse drying effect which can irritate and flake dry skin, and so here an electric razor may be the better choice.

How to clean normal to dry skin

Cleansing creams and lotions clean dry to normal facial skin very effectively. They remove stale oil and dirt from your pores without drying your skin.

Massage the cream gently into your skin with your fingertips, using a circular motion away from the center of your face. (Touch the delicate skin surrounding your eyes, very gently and with care. The direction of your fingertips should always be toward your nose, not away.) Work the cream over the skin and into your pores, to lift out the sebum and dirt. When you wipe off the cream with a tissue, you leave a fine film of protective oil on your skin. Depending upon their consistency, cleansing lotions are either massaged over your skin or applied to cotton and wiped on to dissolve grease and remove it with the dirt.

As a general rule, creams are emulsions of oils and water. The lotions usually contain varying amounts of alcohol in addition to the oil and water. In order to advertise and differentiate one brand from another, manufacturers may add other ingredients to their creams and lotions which often have only marginal benefits, if any. Because of the wide variety and differing strengths of these preparations, read the usage directions carefully to determine the skin type for which it was designed, and choose one made by a reputable firm. A fifty-two-year-old friend of mine with dry skin has been using only cleansing cream on his face for years. His complexion looks twenty.

Optional cleaning methods

Steam treatments help clean out the pores of normal and oily skins; however, their use is optional for skin care. The moist heat opens your pores, and the increased perspiration flow unclogs them and carries out old grease, dirt, and other impurities. Wipe your face gently with a tissue after a treatment and you'll be surprised how much dirt comes out of your pores which you thought looked perfectly clean.

If you have an acne or blackhead problem, a steam treatment may help you. Place one of the various commercial preparations or a few dried camomile flowers in a bowl filled with boiling water. Hold your face over the water and cover your head and the bowl with a towel. Steam for three to five minutes. It's very easy and might be just the answer to your problem.

Face masks—trick or treat? A controversial but invigorating cleaning method is the face mask. Applied wet to your face, the mask supposedly opens your pores, draws out dirt and oil, and then contracts to close your pores again. The entire process takes from five to twenty minutes and leaves your face feeling tight—so tight you might want to apply a moisturizing cream to loosen up your smile. I personally feel that if men keep their skin well cleaned with the methods outlined previously, the main benefits of a face mask would be psychological ones.

Face masks come in all strengths depending upon skin type and sensitivity, so read the usage directions very carefully. Why not get the feel of a mask by whipping up one that you can make from ingredients in your own kitchen?

> Mix one egg yolk with a few drops of lemon juice and a dash of olive oil. Blend well and spread the mixture evenly over your face omitting the skin around your eyes. Relax for about twenty minutes and feel this mask on your skin. Remove with water.
>
> *or*
>
> Beat together an egg white and a teaspoon of olive oil until smooth. Apply as above and remove after twenty minutes with a warm, wet towel.

If you have time before going out some evening, you might try a mask—you'll feel loaded for bear.

3. Tone your skin

When you tone your skin, you're stimulating it and firming it up. You do this by splashing on cold water or by slapping your face with an astringent. Chilling your skin with cold water or by the rapid evaporation of alcohol closes the pores which you've opened while bathing, showering, or shaving, and makes your skin feel tight. The physical action of slapping or rubbing your face increases blood circulation to make your skin feel healthy and glowing.

Toning completes your cleaning process by closing the pores, and it has a beneficial physical and psychological effect on you. Incorporate it in your daily grooming routine if you aren't doing so already.

4. Moisturize your skin

Adding this step to your daily regimen may be the single most productive thing you can do to make your complexion more attractive and keep it looking younger.

It's the moisture in your skin that keeps it soft and supple. You often hear about the beautiful, radiant look an expectant mother gets. This is fact, not fiction. In pregnancy, the increased estrogen hormone levels cause a woman's skin to retain more water which usually results in a noticeable improvement in her skin's appearance. Up to a point, the more moisture you can retain in your skin, the softer and plumper it will feel, the less noticeable its tiny wrinkles, and the more youthful its appearance.

After thoroughly cleaning and toning your skin, a moisturizer puts back a thin film of oil. As oil and water don't mix, this film acts as a barrier to trap some of the moisture in your skin which would otherwise have evaporated into the air. Oily skin doesn't need a moisturizer because it retains enough moisture to stand up well to the effects of age. But experts agree that a moisturizer can benefit the appearance of dry and normal skin which would otherwise deteriorate and wrinkle faster with age.

Use a pure, natural oil or one of the many commercial moisturizing creams and lotions which consist basically of a light emulsion of oil and water with or without a perfume and additives. You don't have to use much. Remember, it's the amount of moisture in your skin that counts, not the thickness and fragrance of the oil on it.

How to apply a moisturizer

After cleaning and toning your skin, put a small dab of moisturizer under each cheek and in the center of your forehead. Gently smooth in the cream using a V pattern from the chin to your ears and from the bridge of your nose to the ears. Use an M pattern on your forehead, massaging from the eyebrows up to your hairline and back down along your sideburns. Tissue any greasy-looking areas. With a little experience you'll find the right amount of moisturizer for your particular skin type. The entire process shouldn't take more than twenty seconds and will leave your face feeling soft and smooth.

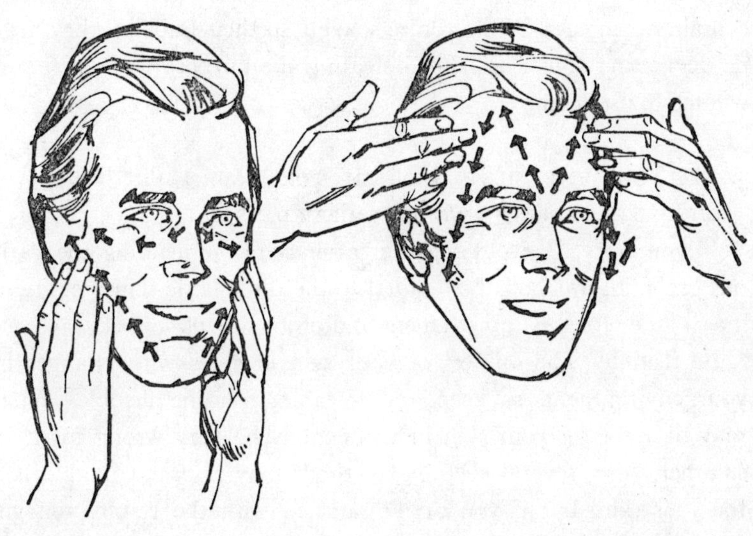

Remember these three basic rules: 1. Smooth the moisturizer gently into your skin taking care not to touch the delicate "bag" skin around your eyes. 2. You need only a very little oil to create the desired film barrier. 3. Avoid overuse, which will give you an unwanted greasy look.

DON'T FORGET YOUR BODY

Chronic, dry body skin or skin that has been exposed to a drying environment (such as on vacation when the sun, wind, and water get at your entire body) should be moisturized to help keep it soft and inhibit flaking. This will also help you keep your suntan longer.

Use a bath oil in the tub or smooth on a light natural oil after bathing. Again, it's the moisture trapped in your skin, not the oil on it, that makes your skin soft and pliable, so don't overdo the oil.

Beware of bath foams and other luxurious bath preparations that contain detergents. While you're soaking in their bubbles, they may be degreasing your skin, thus defeating the purpose for which you wanted to use them.

5. FOLLOW THE BEST REGIMEN FOR YOUR SKIN AND YOU SHOULD SEE RESULTS WITHIN THIRTY DAYS!

In summary, I've put together a chart recommending the various grooming methods best suited to the three basic skin types. Use it as a guide for the improvement and protection of your skin.

Be flexible. The oiliness of your skin changes with changes in your environment, so keep your cleaning routine flexible. What may be right for your skin in winter may be very wrong for it in summer. Also, several cleaning methods may appear equally good for your skin, but if you aren't satisfied with the results you get from one, switch to another.

"NOURISH" YOUR SKIN FROM WITHIN

This is a very sticky subject but one that deserves discussion if you don't want to waste your time and effort on things that won't benefit your skin. To the dermatologist, "nourishing" the skin means feeding it with raw materials to make new, healthy skin cells, but to the cosmetician, it generally means making the skin soft and smooth. Keep this distinction in mind when evaluating manufacturers' claims for their preparations.

Where does your skin get its nourishment?

Your skin gets its nutrients and oxygen from the blood within, although some oxygen comes from outside. Therefore, the nourishment and consequent health of your skin depends upon your diet and the internal functions and over-all health of your body.

Can cosmetic preparations nourish your skin?

Commercially advertised products applied to the outside of your skin can clean it, contract it, and help it retain moisture to keep soft and smooth, but no cosmetic rubbed on the skin has been proved to stop aging or to rejuvenate the skin through its pores.

The outer surface of your skin is dead tissue and thus incapable of being nourished or brought back to life by the application of creams or anything else. Your skin acts as a protective sheath, and only few fatty substances in emulsion with water (like lanolin) can penetrate the outer layer, and only then by being diligently rubbed into the sebaceous and sweat glands. These glands don't store this material but excrete it back onto your skin's surface or else pass it through their thin walls into the bloodstream.

Very few additives can be combined with this fatty emulsion to penetrate into the bloodstream, and, in any case, anything introduced into the blood from external sources without a doctor's prescription cannot be of sufficient concentration to have any significant effect. At this time I know of no additives you can buy over the counter that will benefit the health of male skin in this manner.

RECOMMENDED SKIN CARE REGIMENS

	DRY SKIN	NORMAL SKIN	OILY SKIN
SHAVING:	*Dry shave*	*Dry or wet shave*	*Wet shave*
BATH/ SHOWER:	*Shower:* If not available, take a quick bath in warm, not hot, water. or *Bath:* If you add oil to the water or apply it to your body after.	*Shower or bath:* Add water softener if needed.	*Bath:* Add water softener if needed.
ALTERNATE CLEANSING METHOD*:	*Cleansing cream or lotion* *Soap:* Use sparingly a very mild brand recommended by your doctor or pharmacist.	*Cleansing cream or lotion* *Soap:* Regular, super-fatted, or deodorant Astringent†	*Soap:* Super-fatted, detergent, medicated or liquid brand, or deodorant Astringent†

TONING:	*Mild astringent*† Apply sparingly to remove film left from cleansing cream and soap scum. Don't use regularly if you use soap and your skin feels too tight. plus *Cold water:* Splash face 12 times and towel, leaving some moisture.	*Regular astringent*† Apply sparingly to remove film left from cleansing cream or soap scum. plus *Cold water:* Splash face 12 times and towel, leaving some moisture.	*Strong astringent*† Apply freely to remove soap scum and further degrease skin. plus *Cold water:* Splash face 12 times.
MOISTURIZING:	*Moisturizing cream.*	*Moisturizing cream or lotion.*	*Not usually needed.*

* Only one of the alternate cleansing methods should be used at a time.

† If you use an astringent to cleanse your face, don't use it a second time in the toning process.

BEWARE OF PROBLEMS AND DISEASES THAT CAN MAR YOUR SKIN

Many skin problems and diseases come from viruses, bacteria, fungus, and the reaction of your body to various internal stimuli. Like most diseases of the body, the longer you allow them to develop, the more difficult they become to cure. At the first symptoms of a problem skin condition, take action and/or consult your doctor or dermatologist. There is no point in taking chances with such a visible part of your appearance.

Most skin diseases have nothing to do with improper diet, nutritional deficiences, or digestion. Shortages of protein, carbohydrate, fat, or vitamins cause none of the common skin complaints. Constipation often bears the blame for a bad complexion, but skin diseases don't arise from an accumulation of hypothetical "impurities" in the blood which can be relieved by using the toilet more often. In liver diseases, like jaundice, the skin turns yellow only because the pigment normally excreted through the bowels spills over into your blood and tinges your eyeballs and skin.

Nobody likes to kiss a pimple

A common group of skin diseases (called papulopustular) cause skin eruptions in the form of papules and pustules. A papule is a small, somewhat pointed bump of skin, usually inflamed but without pus. When pus collects, it becomes a pustule or the common pimple. Many diseases fall within this group: acne, rosacea, various types of folliculitis, mila, and the second stage of syphilis (discussed in Chapter 16).

ACNE VULGARIS

Acne vulgaris certainly lives up to its vulgar name and afflicts the majority of white adolescents and young adults. Older men may experience flare-ups of acne due to stress, emotional upset, or a change in climate. Blacks seldom suffer from it, and only eunuchs seem completely immune, but few men would swap a ball to stop a pimple.

It should come as no surprise that acne arises neither through lack of sexual experience nor from masturbation, but its roots do lie in sex. Acne results from your skin's overreaction to stimulation by male hormones. It has been said that the horniest little boys are the pimpliest ones—the same goes for girls.

The cause of acne

With the approach of puberty, increased levels of male hormones stimulate the sebaceous glands which overreact, enlarge, and produce excessive amounts of sebum. The follicules and pores through which this sebum flows become clogged with a waxy plug called a comedo. If closed at the top and not exposed to air, the comedo is a **whitehead.** If open to the air, its contents oxidize and turn black forming a **blackhead** (this has nothing to do with dirt). Unable to reach the surface of the skin through the comedones, the sebum ruptures the sides of the follicules and inflames the surrounding dermis, creating papules. Initially skin-colored, as they become more inflamed they turn red, and pus collects to form pimples. The white blood cells make the pus in trying to subdue the inflammation in the dermis.

Acne papules and pustules usually appear on the face, chest, and back. The problem runs its inevitable course for some years until the skin loses its sensitivity to the hormone stimulation, sebum production falls, and the problem clears up. Acne vulgaris leaves little pits in the skin, sometimes referred to as enlarged pores. The more severe the case, the greater the scarring.

How to fight pimples

Your main weapon in controlling and getting rid of pimples is keeping your skin as free from oil as possible. Cleanse it thoroughly and frequently with special sulfur or medicated soaps and lotions and detergent bars (if very greasy). You must remove all excess sebum and loosen and open comedones to stop pimples from forming. Teen-agers suffering this problem should wash their face thoroughly at least four times a day. Battery-operated facial brushes and gritty soaps can be used to deep-clean pores and loosen the comedones.

Keep hair short. Keep your scalp and hair especially clean, and your hair cut short and brushed away from the face. Oil from the hair and scalp runs down over your face, which is one reason why long-haired men have greater acne problems than their cropped brothers.

What about sun? Exposure to sunlight and the ultraviolet rays often, but not necessarily, helps reduce acne by decreasing the amount of oil in your skin. In severe cases, antibiotics sometimes help stop the sebum trapped in the skin from breaking down into fatty acids which irritate skin, but cleaning represents your most effective defense.

Diet. No really convincing evidence exists to prove that eating starch and such foods as chocolate, nuts, sweets, and fats causes or worsens the average case of acne. Each country seems to blame a different type of food for this condition. As he knows your personal medical history, your doctor can best advise you on a diet.

ROSACEA

DOES HE HAVE IT, OR IS HE DRUNK?

Rosacea chiefly attacks middle-aged people (only occasionally the young) on their forehead, cheeks, chin, and nose. It produces an inflammation of the skin which appears in the form of a red flush of varying degrees from which emerge papules and pustules. Severe rosacea can make your nose redden and swell, which is one of the reasons people unjustly attribute it to alcoholic overindulgence.

The skin of the face reddens noticeably with the consumption of hot drinks, alcohol, spicy foods, and a warm environment. It would seem a Mexican vacation most inadvisable for men suffering this problem. Unlike acne, rosacea has no close association with hormone stimulation, has no blackheads, and leaves no permanent scars.

Treatment often consists of applying sulfur lotions and creams. Severe forms of the disease are difficult to cure, so consult your doctor if symptoms appear.

MILA

White or yellowish beadlike structures lying just under the skin surface are called mila. They usually form spontaneously around the eyes and upper cheek. Mila can be easily picked out by the doctor.

INGROWN HAIR

Papules and pustules commonly result from ingrown hair. This happens when the shaved end of the beard re-enters the skin, continues to grow, and becomes imbedded there. Don't mistake this condition for acne.

When removing an ingrown hair, make sure to sterilize the surrounding skin and your needle or other instrument with alcohol. Depending upon the size and severity of the break you've made in your skin, apply disinfectant and/or a bandage to remove the chance of secondary infection.

BOILS

They'll never appear on your feet

Boils are large oversized pustules which swell painfully, peak and discharge pus after several days. They heal leaving a small round scar. Boils occur only around hairs, never on the hairless palms and soles of your feet.

Bacteria living on your skin and the lining of your nostrils cause boils. As their numbers greatly increase when a boil discharges on the skin, never squeeze it because you'll spread the bacteria, increasing your chances of reinfection. It also opens the wound to secondary infection which could lead to blood poisoning.

Injections of antibiotics may help clear up a boil, but don't affect the bacteria on the skin surface, and so they may fail to stop further boils from occurring. Aside from applying antibiotic and medicated creams to the infection itself, use germicidal creams, powders, shampoos, and soaps to destroy as many of the harmful bacteria on your skin, nose, and hair as possible.

Clothing and bed linen (particularly pillowcases) which come in contact with boils should be changed frequently and washed or dry-cleaned to prevent reinfection. People sometimes blame general ill health or poor diet for causing boils, but apart from diabetes, which encourages various kinds of infection, few constitutional upsets can be blamed for this skin eruption. Concentrate on getting the bacteria.

HERPES

Strike again

Many men regularly suffer from this unattractive infection because, even though in good health, it's always skulking about their skin waiting to strike at the most inopportune times.

A very common viral infection, herpes simplex more often attacks adults than children. The initial infection probably occurs in infancy and heals spontaneously. The virus remains dormant on your skin for years and attacks when conditions suit it best, such as a rise in body temperature, exposure to unaccustomed amounts of sunshine, extreme fatigue, or a general lowering of the body's resistance to infection. Herpes is a recurrent infection, generally appearing in the same area over and over again.

It usually strikes at the skin around the lips, but can hit elsewhere on the body including the genitals—both inhibiting places from the standpoint of sex. The attack consists of itchy, red papules which swell and blister, often being replaced by crusting. The problem usually clears up without scarring in a week or two.

This condition doesn't respond well to treatment and usually continues its inevitable course. Proper care, however, may restrict the duration of the attack. Don't spread and prolong the infection by touching or scratching the problem area. Apply alcohol or astringents frequently during the day. If you suspect dirty work afoot, keep the threatened area dosed with after-shave lotion and cologne even before concrete symptoms appear. Often, bathing the infected area with salt water helps. Look for the factor causing your herpes and try to avoid it in the future.

SHINGLES

Herpes zoster, better known as shingles, is another common but more serious and painful viral infection affecting one or more of your sensory nerves as well as your skin. Shingles characteristically starts with sensitivity or pain in a localized area of your skin. Discomfort may occur before any visible change in the skin. Within a day or two you'll notice redness and some swelling followed by blisters. The blisters fill with a watery fluid and may burst, usually hemorrhaging to form blood scabs. Unless the infection is severe, the eruption usually lasts about ten days or so then improves, leaving circular scars. Unlike herpes simplex, second attacks from herpes zoster are infrequent.

No effective treatment exists for shingles, and the infection takes its course. Your main objective is to relieve your pain with prescribed analgesics and, if more comfortable, to protect the sensitive area with padded gauze. Men with shingles often feel ill and may need bed rest. You most certainly want to consult your doctor if this disease strikes.

WARTS

Call the witch doctor

Skin has probably had more experience with the common wart and its variants than any of the other viral infections. Viral warts generally appear on the exposed parts of your body like the hands and fingers, but the virus can be inoculated into other areas by scratching or through open wounds. You often contact warts on your feet from others with the same condition in swimming pools and bathrooms or sports grounds and gymnasiums.

The common wart represents somewhat of a medical mystery in that if left untreated, it will often disappear in a year or two, but frequently can be induced to leave earlier by suggestion by applying harmless, inactive creams and a little mumbo jumbo. Warts can also be destroyed physically. Because of the wide variety of warts and the many different remedies depending upon age, location, etc., consult your doctor for help with this infection.

PSORIASIS

Psoriasis is a common scaling condition which occurs most often on the scalp, elbows, and knees. The scales look silvery and hard, and when scraped away, the skin underneath sometimes exudes a clear watery liquid. In scale-free areas, the skin looks smooth, dry, and glistening.

Psoriasis is a mystery. It stems from a malformation in the cell structure of the epidermis and is usually inherited. The condition may remain dormant for long periods and then suddenly become active in times of strain and emotional stress. Treatment seems an individual thing. Although it can't be eliminated, cortisone often suppresses the worst aspects of psoriasis. Tar and sulfur compounds and exposure to sun fall on the list of possible treatments.

CHAPTER 4

Suntan: The Beautiful People's Dilemma

Most of us regard a suntan as the mark of the healthy, athletic man or the wealthy hedonist basking on his yacht or in his seaside villa. In London, New York, or Paris one automatically assumes a man tanned out of season is one of the "beautiful people" we hear so much about and has the wealth to afford long vacations on the ski slopes or in the equatorial sun. But ironically, the long-range effects of too much sun can turn a beautiful people into a very wrinkled, prematurely old one. Why not find a new status symbol which lets you have fun and stay youthful-looking at the same time?

THE IDEAL TAN

From the standpoint of preserving youthful, good-looking skin, the perfect tan is practically no tan at all. But as a brown body seems to give us a psychological lift and an appealing appearance by today's standards, you've got to reach a compromise.

On this premise, the ideal tan for Caucasian skin should be an even and over-all darkening of skin color to a medium, golden-brown, or light bronze hue (not a very deep hue) obtained without burning or discomfort. Your skin should remain smooth and soft, not dry and flaky.

Some men will be able to achieve this ideal very easily and should avoid the temptation to go darker and risk skin damage. Others, because of skin sensitivity, shouldn't attempt it, and must be content with only a slight browning or glow to their skin.

HOW SUN AFFECTS YOUR BODY

First of all, rather than being healthy, tanned skin is damaged skin trying to protect itself. When exposed to the sun's ultraviolet rays, a chemical reaction in your skin stimulates the production of pigment (melanin) which darkens your skin as a defense against further penetration by the ultraviolet rays.

Chronic overexposure, so typical with sun worshipers and northerners who've resettled in sunny places, results in skin degeneration. Your skin will age prematurely, reduce its oil production, dry out, and lose its elasticity. It thickens to become leathery and wrinkled. If you have any doubts, just look at the complexion of all the expatriates living in Ibiza and Majorca.

Constant exposure to sun can fleck the skin with brown patches and plays a part in causing common types of easily cured skin cancer. Don't panic; most of us aren't exposed to enough sun to get into this difficulty.

Let's not forget our old "friend" sunburn. Technically it's a superficial inflammation of your skin caused from exposure to ultraviolet rays. A first-degree burn has a slight reddening several hours after exposure without itching or burning sensations. Overexposure produces the very painful third- and fourth-degree burns which are destructive to your skin tissue and result in peeling.

Finally, long periods of sun-gazing can cause a degeneration of the retina which could lead to permanent bad eyesight. Although not proved, some researchers suspect that sunbathing with closed, but unprotected, eyes may eventually encourage deterioration of the retina, and so they advocate that you cover your eyes with dark-lensed sunglasses or some other device. Why take chances?

But there must be some benefits from the sun!

There are some benefits from sunning yourself, but primarily they're the short-term cosmetic and psychological benefits of looking and feeling healthy. And, believe it or not, it encourages sex.

As summer approaches with longer daylight hours, more ultraviolet radiation strikes your eyes. This has a stimulating effect on your sex glands. As a side reaction, the glands stimulate the production of melanin, so your entire body darkens a bit. It would happen even if you were covered from head to toe in a suit of lead. As an extreme example, take the cockerel. If you were to make him wear dark glasses and so cut off the sun from his eyes, his comb, which attracts the hens, wouldn't turn red but remain green. So, you see, the old saying that "in spring a young man's fancy turns to thoughts of love" is quite true, thanks to the sun.

The ultraviolet rays also have a germicidal effect on your skin and so help fight fungal infections and the bacterial causes of some scalp and dandruff conditions. By drying the skin, the sun may have a seasonal therapeutic effect on acne. Your skin makes vitamin D when exposed to sunlight, but this is of little importance as you can pick up enough of this vitamin from a normal, balanced diet.

HOW TO GET A GOOD SUNTAN (IN THE SHORTEST POSSIBLE TIME)

Acquiring a good tan which you can enjoy while you're on vacation instead of after you leave depends upon a delicate balance of three obvious factors: the sensitivity of your skin, how you expose it to the sun, and the protective lotions you use. It's stupid to plunk a white, oiled body down on the beach for hours the first day only to burn, peel, and have it start all over again. It's stupid, but most of us do it and so don't really end up with the tan we want until the last few days of the vacation. If you stick to the following regimen, you should get a good tan in the shortest possible time without discomfort or damage to your skin.

Prevacation

1. **Condition your skin** as early in the year as possible by exposing it to the sun while it's at a safe low angle. As summer approaches, adapt your exposure times to the increasing intensity of the sun, gradually building a light base tan before taking on long doses of more intense vacation sun.
2. Alternately, **use a sunlamp** at home for a few weeks before going on vacation. Although I've yet to see a good tan produced solely by an ultraviolet lamp, they can be helpful in preparing your skin for future exposure to the sun and for prolonging a natural suntan.

There are two common types of ultraviolet sunlamps for home use: the glass bulb lamp used mainly for tanning and the hot quartz lamp for both tanning and germicidal purposes. Most certainly follow the directions accompanying any sunlamp, but in general, lamps should be placed about thirty inches from your skin to get the proper concentration of tanning rays. If placed closer (up to twelve inches), you risk possible skin tissue destruction. For average skin, start by exposing yourself for about two or three minutes and gradually work up to around ten minutes.

Warning: At least one day should elapse between exposures, and always wear goggles to protect your eyes from the ultraviolet rays.

3. If available, try a series of **professional ultraviolet treatments** at a salon. They more effectively lay down a protective foundation over your entire body. Often exposure time can run as high as twenty minutes because here you have the benefit of constant observation by experts who can judge your skin's reaction to the lamp rays.

During vacation

It comes as no surprise to you that men with fair skin (usually accompanied by light blue, hazel, or gray eyes and light or red hair) have trouble tanning. Their thinner skin is extremely sensitive to the burning rays and should have less exposure and more protection than men with darker eyes, hair, and skin. In some cases tanning may be impossible. One of the advantages of maturity is that older men tan faster and darker than their juniors.

1. **Exposure:** The more atmosphere and cloud cover the sun's rays must penetrate before reaching your skin, the less potent their effect. The low angle of the sun in the mornings and afternoons forces the rays to pass diagonally through more atmosphere than when directly overhead at noon. Therefore, start your tan by exposing your body for an hour in the morning and an hour in the afternoon when the sun lies low. Cover up and go touring or sit in the shade during the fierce midday sun.

Increase your skin's exposure gradually. Take particular care of those areas that get more intense exposure like your nose and shoulders, and those areas that seldom see light like the tops of your feet, ankles, backs of knees, and, for the nudists, the genitals. If you ever get a sunburn there, you'll know it!

Skiers, beware. Take into account your altitude and the sun's reflection when planning your exposure time. The higher you climb above sea level, the thinner the atmosphere, the less the air pollution, and the more intense the sun. Also use extra protection against the ultraviolet rays reflected from water and snow. They greatly increase the tanning and burning effects of the sun.

Finally, remember that ultraviolet rays are known as the cold, invisible rays. On hazy days when the sun's warmth is blotted out, the ultraviolet rays can penetrate through to burn your skin even though your body feels cool. Use just as much caution as you would in brilliant sunshine.

2. **Suntan preparations:** Frequently apply a suntan preparation to protect your skin from overexposure to the ultraviolet rays and to keep it from dehydrating. Select one for your degree of skin sensitivity and the length of exposure.

In reality almost all tanning preparations should be called "antiburn" or "sun-protection" products because that's precisely their function. Only about 2 to 3 per cent of all the sun's rays cause your skin to tan or burn. Unfortunately, the rays that tan your skin overlap with the rays that burn it, and the burning rays are the most active tanners. This poses real problems for the manufacturers. The ideal product would "screen" out just enough harmful rays to minimize the risk of burning while allowing enough through for good tanning in the fastest possible time. Considering varying sensitivities of skin, you'll have to agree the manufacturers' task is virtually impossible, so you've got to use your common sense.

Here's a good tip. Some ethical preparations for very sensitive or a baby's skin screen out virtually 100 per cent of all ultraviolet rays and so give almost complete protection. You could lie on the beach for hours and get little more than a blush of color. Keep one of these preparations on hand for use on any skin areas that might inadvertently get burned, like your nose or the arm resting out the car window. This will enable you to continue taking the sun without complicating the smaller burned areas. (Ask your doctor or pharmacist for his recommendation.)

Unfortunately, you have little to guide you buying the sun preparations most effective for your needs because they all claim basically the same things, "a fast, rich, glorious tan." Price can't be relied upon as an indication of effectiveness. A study conducted in 1972 by the London newspaper the *Evening Standard* showed that some of the cheaper brands were far better against sunburn than some of their ritzier competitors from cosmetic houses priced as much as eight times higher. As the formulations of these preparations can change from one year to the next, consult consumer protection publications like *Consumer Report* and *Which?* for their evaluations.

Some preparations actually do "tan" your skin. They contain chemicals which, regardless of sun, interact with your skin surface to produce a superficial color lasting about a week. But don't be fooled into thinking your artificial tan will protect you. Until your skin develops its own natural protective tan, you can get a whopper of a burn.

3. **Sunglasses:** Wear dark green or gray sunglasses when in the sun. While sunbathing with your eyes closed, cover your lids with something to protect your eyes from possible harm. Never look directly at, or squint at, the sun. (See pages 104–5 on selecting sunglasses.)

4. **Après sun:** Upon leaving the sun, bathe in warm, not hot, water to remove perspiration, salt, and suntan oil. Then apply a natural oil or moisturizer all over your body to help your skin retain mositure and keep it from drying and flaking off its tanned outer tissue.

Keeping your tan

1. After your vacation, continue to expose your skin to the sun or use a sunlamp. Don't overdo the lamp. Because of its strength,

you might burn or overly dry your skin, thus encouraging it to peel or flake.

2. It's quite true that you can wash your tan down the drain by loosening and removing skin tissue. Take brief showers, not hot baths, and continue to apply a light oil or moisturizer to your body (particularly your face) to keep your skin smooth and stop your tan from flaking off.

THE PROBLEM OF PHOTOSENSITIVE SKIN

The chances of you developing photosensitive skin are small but increasing with the increased use of toiletries, fragrances, and some drugs. Men over forty who go in for developing deep suntans run a greater risk. I've known several in this category who've had real problems.

Photosensitive skin overreacts to the action of radiant energy, especially light. There are two basic types: phototoxicity and the less common, photoallergic reaction.

Phototoxicity occurs when your skin overreacts to intense sunlight (even through windows, occasionally from fluorescent lights) because of some offending agent which you've taken internally or applied externally. This combination usually produces an exaggerated sunburn on those skin surfaces most often bared to the sun (your hands, face, and chest) and can occur from minutes to hours after exposure to light. The reaction may even strike while you're fully clothed, not just while sunbathing.

Drugs that may cause phototoxicity are: antibiotics of the tetracycline family (chlortetracycline, the big offender, often being recommended for acne); sulfur drugs and sulfur derivatives like thiazine diuretics and oral hypoglycemic agents sometimes used as substitutes for insulin by mild diabetics; sulfonamides, often prescribed for infections of the urinary tract; and tranquilizers of the phenothiazine type such as Thorazine and Stelazine. These tranquilizers may also cause your eyes to become photosensitive, producing irritation, tearing, and low tolerance to strong light.

Photoallergic reactions, as the name implies, depend upon the individual's allergic susceptibility to various substances usually applied externally. The reaction to some chemicals may be an itchy red rash (like poison ivy) appearing from one to three days after exposure to sun. The essential oils in some perfumes and after-shave lotions might bring on a spotty brown skin discoloration that can last a long time. After a day on the beach, a girl friend of mine developed brown patches everywhere she applied her perfume—a fascinating revelation. It's best to wear only tanning oil when exposing your body to the sun.

Possible photosensitizers are: bactericidal chemicals often found in deodorant soaps; oils like citron, sandlewood, lavender, and bergamot; tar shampoos and detergents; sunscreens in tanning preparations; and even handling plants like ragweed, parsley, fennel, carrots, parsnips, and figs.

Treating photosensitive skin usually consists of ridding yourself of the photosensitizers and staying out of the sunlight. A skin reaction may stay with you for some time, even in the absence of the offending agent, and occasionally skin may be left permanently overreactive to sunlight, so those unlucky few had better be prepared to spend their vacations looking at prehistoric drawings in French caves.

CHAPTER 5

Cosmetic Surgery: How It Can Help You

Although you can't expect a toad to change miraculously into a prince charming with just the wave of a surgeon's scalpel, today you can use cosmetic plastic surgery to make yourself a strikingly more handsome and youthful-looking man.

Kurt heads a successful multinational company. His name can usually be found in the guest books of the most attractive hostesses on the Continent and in New York, and he's seldom seen without a young lovely on his arm. Kurt is in his mid-fifties but looks forty. Why? He's had cosmetic surgery done on his eyelids.

Vince Hill, the not-so-young English singer, had his prominent Roman nose reshaped to better fit into the current youthful pop scene.

A young South African businessman had his protruding ears set back against his head for a more serious look. He now runs his own thriving company. The names of the men who have discreetly undergone one form or another of cosmetic surgery would make the best-seller list.

Cosmetic surgery can make you more handsome and shed years from your age by eliminating sagging jowls, deep wrinkles, and bags from under your eyes. Men use it to help protect their jobs from younger-looking competitors on their way up, or just to look and feel a hell of a lot better. Dr. Paul Pickering, a San Diego plastic surgeon, once said, "When you see what a simple face-lift can do for a depressed, out-of-work executive, you've got to be impressed. It changes not only his face, but his whole outlook; gives him new vitality and confidence."

Don't regard plastic surgery as a flippant new medium created solely to rejuvenate and gratify the whims of men and women. Hindus practiced it in 1000 B.C. to reconstruct the severed noses of prisoners and unfaithful wives. Plastic surgery came into a new era of sophistication and technology during the twentieth century because of our desperate need to restore the shattered bodies of the World Wars. As so often happens, the skills acquired in war have benefited us in peace. Today surgeons use the improved techniques in plastic surgery to:

- correct congenital defects such as cleft palates and lips, malformed ears and limbs that used to doom children to lives of mental anguish.
- restore skin and bone damage from burns and accidents. My Yale roommate had his entire skull put back together and his features reformed after a teen-age motorcycle crash near London. Not knowing about the accident, we looked upon him as just another handsome, but slightly mad, Englishman.
- correct defects caused by paralysis, muscle atrophy, and other illnesses.

• alter and improve features of the face and body simply to make their owners more handsome and youthful-looking.

THE IDEAL OF COSMETIC SURGERY

Structurally, the ideal face produced by cosmetic surgery should result in a harmonious relationship of features in both size and shape. There should be no abnormal skin coloration or noticeable scarring to indicate surgery has ever been done.

Ideal eyelid surgery or a face-lift should leave your facial skin firm but supple, free from bags and bulges around the eyes, deep wrinkles, and sagging jowls, cheeks, and chins. Again, no noticeable scarring should be present.

HOW TO DECIDE UPON COSMETIC SURGERY

1. First, should you change your features?

What do you really look like? You'll probably never know. The image you see in the mirror is reversed and at a distorted perspective, and you modify it in your mind by what you think you look like or should look like. Be honest. How often do you think a photograph is a good likeness of yourself? Like most of us, don't you search through the pile to find the one that comes closest to your ideal of a handsome man?

We all have unreal images of ourselves based upon our appearance when we were younger and what we think society considers handsome. Our self-images don't depend so much on visual objectivity, as on our point of view. Men seldom think they look as old, as fat, or as thin as they really are. Fat men consider themselves "muscular" and skinny men, "slim." If you have a negative point of view, the reverse can be true. No matter how handsome, you consider yourself plain, unattractive, or even downright ugly.

Bearing this in mind, approach cosmetic surgery with some caution. Are you correcting a real or imagined disfigurement? Don't undergo surgery to change a minor abnormality which gives your face distinction and character. There may be no cosmetic reason to change any of the features of your face, and yet for some psychological reason you don't like it or want to escape from it. In these cases, doctors often recommend you talk with a psychiatrist to see if your desire for change can't be eased, or they bluntly refuse to perform the surgery.

2. Make sure you really want to be handsome

Psychologically some people rely upon a disfigurement or physical abnormality as a crutch to justify their current life situation. Men can hide behind obesity or an ugly nose as an excuse for their lack of business and social success. Lose the weight or correct the nose and the excuse disappears. Now the newly created handsome man has only himself to blame for his failure or the fact that people don't like him. Some men can't stand this realization.

3. Don't change the wrong features

You may be unhappy with the proportions of your face without knowing exactly why and therefore elect to change the wrong thing. For example, you might think your nose too long when, in fact, by extending your chin your entire face could be brought into perfect balance. In cases like this, always be guided by your surgeon: he knows best what should be done.

4. Get your timing right

Structural changes can be made at almost any time during your adult life if no conflicting medical or health problems exist. The earlier in life an obvious disfigurement can be corrected, the better.

A face-lift or eyelid surgery should be done when the results will be noticeable and satisfy you. The majority of face-lifts are carried out between the ages of forty and fifty-five years. A lift may last five years or longer depending upon your type of skin and your habits of facial expression. An overanimated or frowning face may need earlier secondary surgery.

Because of its relative simplicity, surgery to remove fatty tissue and wrinkles from around the eyes is often done at a much earlier age, particularly among men who depend upon their youth and good looks for their living. Both eyelid operations and face-lifts can be repeated within reasonable limits.

Fortunately, nature comes to the aid of a cosmetic surgeon. The skin of your face heals better with less scarring than the rest of your body. Also, older skin may heal with less visible scarring than young skin. In any event, surgery is performed so that what little scarring exists is hidden to a great extent by natural folds in your skin or covered by hair.

HOW COSMETIC SURGERY WORKS

Many different operations and variations on these operations can be performed to improve the bone structure of your face or to make you look younger. I will deal here with only the most common ones that may be of value to you now or in the future.

Eyelid operations (blepharoplasty)

This operation removes excess skin and fatty tissue from your lower and upper eyelids. By so doing, the surgeon eliminates the "bags" from under and the "bulges" over your eyes as well as the associated age wrinkles.

The lower lid: The surgeon makes his incision (a) just below the margin of your eye and partially down one of your smile lines so your natural skin folds will help hide any minor scars. When peeled back, the skin flap reveals the fatty tissue, which is removed (b). Excess skin is trimmed from the flap, which can then be stitched back into place (c).

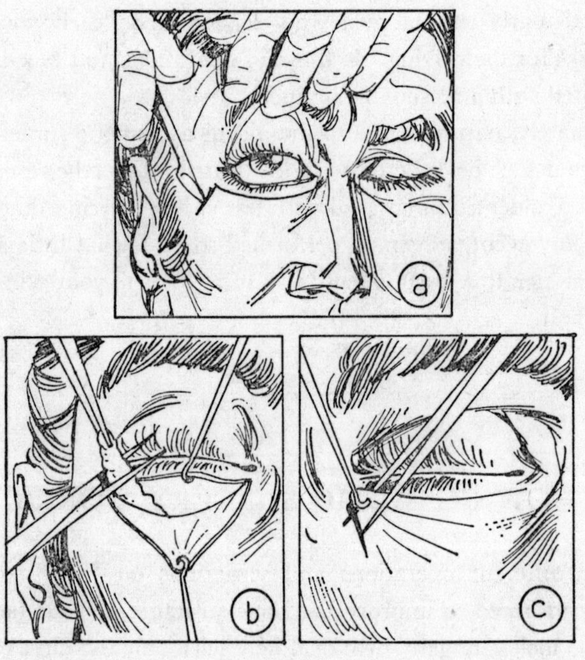

The upper lid: Here the incision runs along the normal crease of your eyelid where it will be covered when your eye is open. As with the lower lid, the skin flap is raised, fatty tissue removed, the flap trimmed and stitched back in place. Care must be taken to leave enough skin to enable your eyelid to close normally over the eye (d).

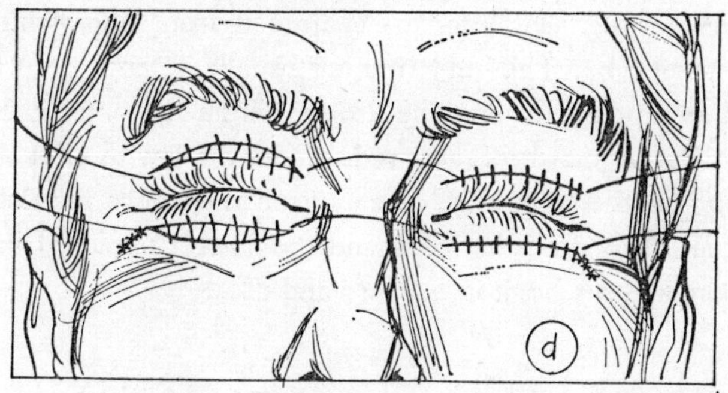

The surgery for upper and lower eyelid operations is relatively simple and usually involves only a day or so in the hospital. When performing both in the same session, it's best to keep your eyes bandaged for at least twelve hours. (Some surgeons prefer no bandages and apply wet compresses.) The stitches can be removed in about four days. The skin around your eyes will be bruised (black and blue), but this discoloration should disappear in two weeks. Initially the minor scars will be pink, but gradually fade in a few months. A three-week "vacation" with dark glasses should see you through without any undue embarrassment.

The cost of each type of eyelid operation runs from $650.

The face-lift

With middle age, skin loses some of its elasticity and your cheeks and neck tend to sag and the folds of skin extending from your nose down around the mouth deepen. The tissue along your jaw appears to fall forward, and your tendency to jowls increases. A face-lift pulls your facial skin up and back toward the hairline, taking up the slack to eliminate much of the jowls, skin folds, and wrinkles. It thus gives your face a firmer, more youthful look.

The incision starts in the region of your temple, runs down the hairline in front of your ear, around the back of the ear, and along the hairline at the nape of your neck (a). Your skin is undermined on a superficial level to separate it from underlying supporting tissue (b). This undermining usually extends only as far forward as a perpendicular line dropped from the outer corner of your eye, but in some cases goes right under the jaw to meet the undermining on the other side. The surgeon then pulls the skin flap upward and back until he has found the correct tension, trims the excess skin, and stitches it in place (c and d).

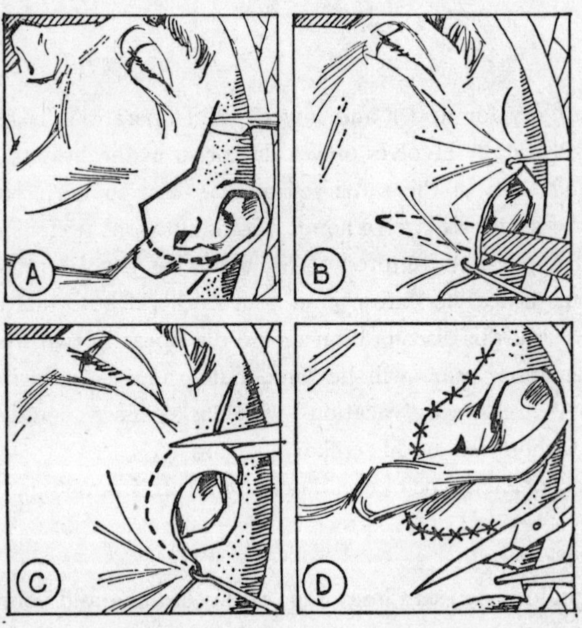

During the next forty-eight hours, any fluids collecting in the undermined areas are drained off and your face kept well bandaged. The fine stitches, not under tension, are usually removed in about three to four days; the last major ones about ten days after the operation. Assuming no complications, all scar lines should fade and puffiness and discoloration subside in about three weeks, leaving you free to go back into circulation after having shed a few years. The cost of this operation can vary between $1,000 and $2,000.

Dermabrasion

Dermabrasion has been used with varying success to remove skin pocked by severe acne or marked by other illnesses and troubles, and to replace it with new skin growth.

A high-speed rotating brush abrades away the offending layers of facial skin. The fluids resulting from this skin removal are absorbed for a few hours and then the face bandaged. It will sting for about a day, after which the bandages are removed to facilitate the crusting that forms over the abraded area. In about five days the crust begins to peel off with the aid of soaking the face in a warm solution. The crust should be completely shed in up to two weeks, leaving a layer of pink new skin.

Aside from the skill of the operator, the success of dermabrasion depends upon the depth and nature of your problem and the reaction of your skin to this type of treatment.

Cosmetic nose surgery (rhinoplasty)

The over-all shape of your nose can be corrected by changing the shape of one or more of its parts:

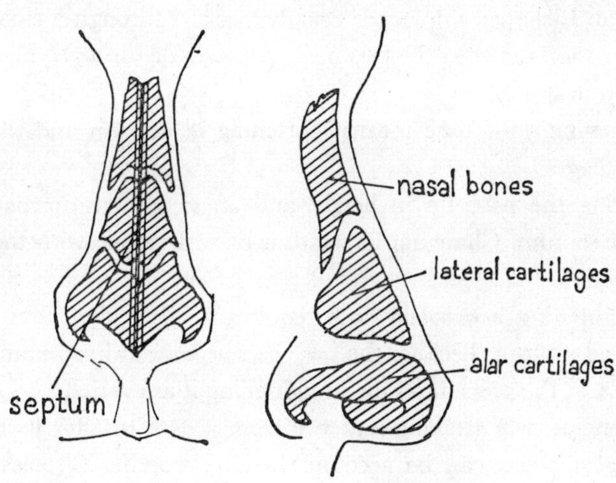

The septum dictates the height and lateral direction of the bridge line of your nose below the nasal bones and helps support the nose tip. As such, it bears the responsibility for the angle of your nose with the face.

The nasal bones extend from your skull and meet the septum in mid line.

The lateral cartilages connect to the nasal bones and septum and extend down the side walls of the nose. These cartilages help maintain the width, height, and length of your nose.

The alar cartilages are supported by the lateral cartilages and fit closely to the septum. They bear most of the responsibility for the shape of your nose tip and could support the tip without help from the septum.

Correcting the bridge line of your nose by removing its "hump" calls for shaving down the nasal bones and trimming the septum and lateral cartilages. To balance the shape after removing the bump, the nose usually has to be thinned and narrowed. This was the type of operation performed on Vince Hill.

Building up a depressed nose requires implanting a small, carefully shaped sliver of bone, cartilage, or hard silicone into a slot prepared in your bridge. If the nose tip needs support as well as the bridge, an L-shaped implant is usually inserted through a small external incision between the two nasal passages or through the lower part of your septum.

Shortening your nose means shortening its septum and the lateral cartilages.

Altering the nose tip in height and angle of elevation is done with the septum. Changing its width is basically done with the alar cartilages.

Straightening a crooked nose requires straightening your nasal bones and septum. Because the nose can be broken in so many different ways, the procedures for straightening it are varied.

In general, when taking material from a nose to alter its shape, the surgical work can be accomplished by working through incisions made inside the nose under local anesthesia. Normal skin, freed from the supporting bone and cartilage which the surgeon is reducing, will contract down to the new shape of the nose without wrinkling and looking baggy.

After nose operations, iced compresses are often used for a day or so to reduce the swelling that normally occurs around your eyes and cheeks. Depending upon the severity of the operation, you must usually remain in the hospital for about three to five days for observation and your bandages checked biweekly until healing is complete, usually in three to four weeks. Some skin discoloration may remain up to three weeks. Most new noses take about six months to reach their final shape. The results are permanent.

The cost of reducing a nose usually runs around $750.

Cosmetic chin surgery

Many men have receding chins which can make their faces look weak, throw their other features out of balance, and contribute to the formation of double chins. To correct this, a silicone bone or cartilage implant can be fitted over their jawbone to extend it forward. The implant can usually be inserted through an incision made inside the mouth to eliminate external scarring; however, some surgeons prefer the external approach through a small incision in a skin crease immediately under the chin. If the jaw is severely receded, more drastic jaw surgery must be undertaken which also takes into consideration the realignment of the patient's bite. This work is often done by dental surgeons.

Ear surgery

I'll bet you don't usually notice another person's ears—unless they are abnormal in some way, and then you can't take your eyes off them. Fortunately, abnormalities ranging from ears that just stick out too far (bat ears) to completely missing ears can be corrected or reconstructed through surgery today with amazing results.

Think of your ear as a thin sandwich of two pieces of skin tightly covering an internal cartilage. It's an amazing structure of curves and buttresses which maintain its shape and stability, which is a fortunate thing for those of you who now wear glasses.

Setting back ears: Protruding ears probably represents the most common ear problem. The corrective operation involves setting them back by the sides of your head, and if missing or too small, reproducing the antihelix ridge to give your ears a more normal shape. The operation is performed on both ears in the same session. The surgeon tackles the worst one first so the more easily corrected ear can be matched to it.

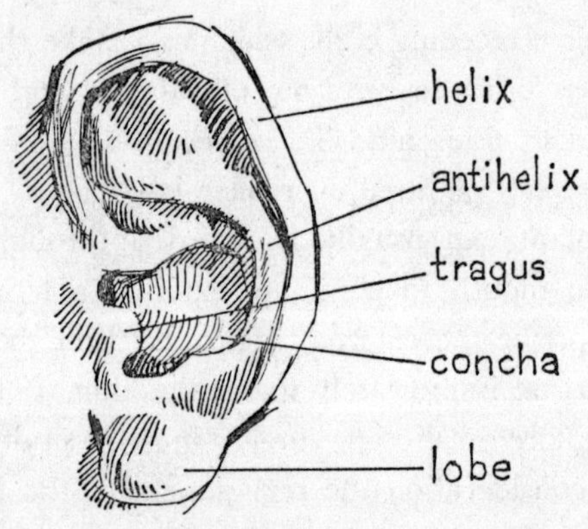

First, the form of the antihelix ridge is marked on the front of your ear and a dye-tipped needle inserted completely through the ear to mark it on the interior cartilage (a). An ellipse of skin is cut away (b). The more your ears protude, the more skin must be removed. The blood vessels are tied.

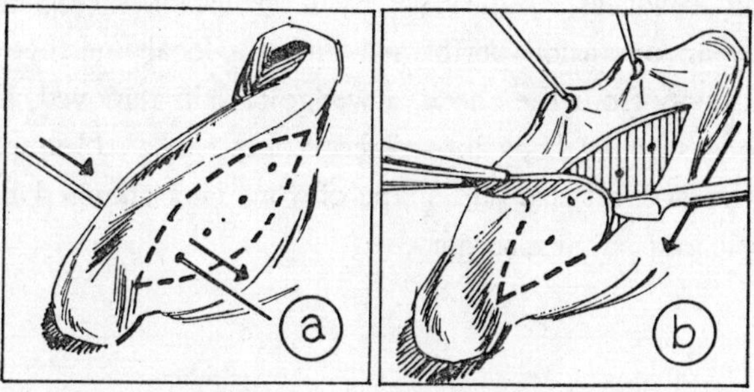

Next an incision is made in the cartilage along the path of the dots marking the antihelix ridge, and the skin on the front of your ear freed from the incision area. A longitudinal strip of cartilage may be cut, excised, or thinned (c). (Some surgeons may simply create the antihelix fold by posterior sutures without treating the cartilage.)

When sufficient cartilage has been removed to allow your ear to lie back comfortably without a tendency to return to its old position, the surgeon stitches together the sides of the elliptical incision in the skin (d). Bandages can be removed after seven days, but the ear should be protected for about two weeks. The cost runs from $650.

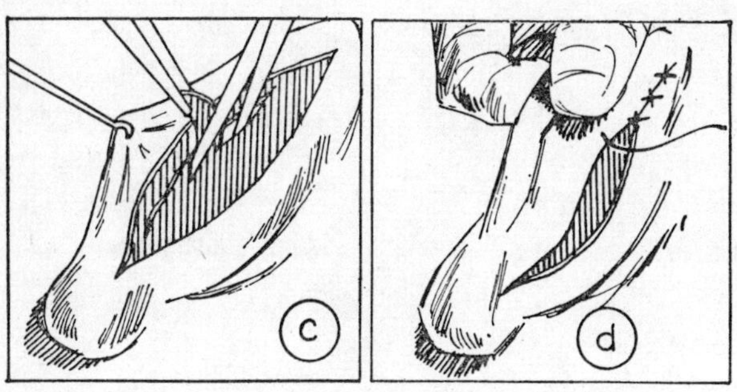

Treating earlobes: Embarrassingly large earlobes can easily be reduced by an operation performed under a local anesthetic. The lobe is cut away from the cheek, a wedge of skin removed, and the reduced lobe stitched back into place. Lobes can also be added to ears and the over-all size and shape of your ears changed by relatively simple and painless surgery.

Chapter 6

Eyesight: How to Preserve and Protect Your Sight

Your life is sight orientated. Almost everything you do depends upon seeing things and reacting to them. About half of all the fibers carrying messages to your brain come from the optic nerves. You should therefore regard your eyes as your most vital sensory organs. It would be tragic to damage or lose them through ignorance and carelessness.

IDEAL EYESIGHT

Perfect sight relies upon the optical proportions of both your eyes being exact so each can focus on an object some twenty feet away without any "accommodative" assistance. Only about one or two people in a hundred between the ages of ten and forty-five can meet this criterion.

The movement of both eyes should be co-ordinated so that their axes remain parallel. Only the ancient Mayan Indians considered crossed eyes as godlike and so tried to encourage deviation between their own eye movements.

Your eyes should be able to distinguish all colors and degrees of light and darkness.

PROBLEMS OF FOCUS AND HOW TO DEAL WITH THEM

Your eyes function like a camera. Rays of light reflected from an object pass through the transparent **cornea** and **lens** of your eye, which focus them into a sharp image on the surface of your light-sensitive **retina.** The convex shape of the cornea does most of the

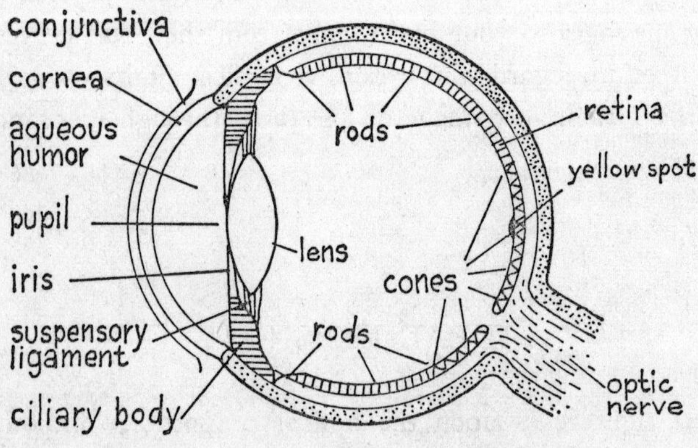

focusing, but your lens does the necessary "fine tuning." To do this, the muscles of the **ciliary body** tighten and relax to alter the convex shape of the lens. This alteration is called accommodation.

The retina contains over a hundred million light receptors (**cones** and **rods**), which convert the patterns of color and light into nerve impulses and send them through the **optic nerve** to your brain. A **yellow spot** lies in the retina directly opposite your pupil. Its center (the **fovea centralis**) is the size of a pinhead and gives you your most acute vision. That's why you see things more clearly when looking straight ahead.

Unfortunately, while physics demands exact dimensions, biology does not. Just as other parts of your body vary in size and contour, so your eyeball usually varies from ideal optical proportions. This creates difficulties in focusing images on your retina.

Longsightedness (hypermetropia)

About 50 per cent of the people in Western races suffer some degree of longsightedness because their eyeballs are slightly shorter than the ideal. Thus reflected light from distant objects comes to a perfect focus behind the retina, leaving only semiformed, hazy images for the rods and cones to pass on to the brain. The lens can compensate for this through accommodation so that a longsighted

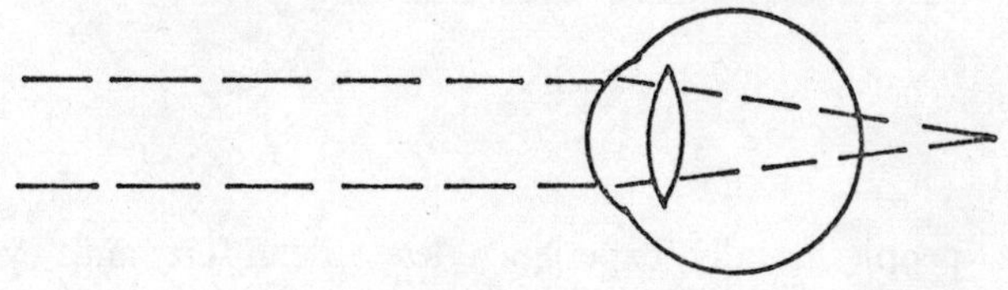

man sees distant objects clearly; however, he must exert greater effort and strain to bring close objects into focus than people with perfect vision.

Longsighted men often develop headaches and dull pain around their eyes and eyebrows. After doing close visual work for some time, they may suffer temporary blurred vision. Eyestrain may result in the form of bloodshot eyes, red edges of the eyelids, frowning, facial twitchings, and, perhaps, a feeling of nausea and depression. If the degree of longsightedness is so great that no amount of accommodation can help, distant objects will be unrecognizable.

Shortsightedness (myopia)

Some 15 to 20 per cent of Western people suffer shortsightedness because their eyeballs tend to be longer than the ideal. Distant objects appear blurred because they come into focus before reaching the retina. Unlike longsightedness, the lens can't accommodate to correct this focus problem and so the eye will only be able to see clearly those objects closer to it. A slight improvement in distant focusing can be obtained by narrowing the eyelids and lowering the eyebrows—a characteristic expression of nearsighted people.

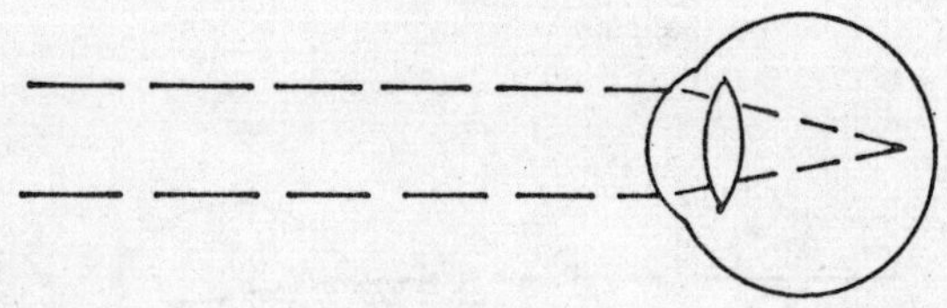

Myopic people usually experience less discomfort and eyestrain than those with longer vision.

Small degrees of longsightedness may go undetected until the age of thirty-five or forty, but myopia usually begins to show at three or four years. This condition tends to increase gradually through adolescence, after which it usually remains more or less stationary. In rare cases it continues to worsen with age, leading to a serious impairment of vision.

Astigmatism

Astigmatism results from an unequal radius of the cornea's surface curvature (shaped more like the bowl of a spoon than a circular dome) and to a lesser degree from unequal curved surfaces of the lens. Regardless of the distance of an object, the cornea and lens can't bend, or refract, all the light rays entering the eye to the same degree and so fail to bring them together into a single focus.

No amount of accommodation can overcome this problem, which gives somewhat distorted and indistinct vision. Objects may appear elongated, circles become ovals, parts of the same letters blur while others are clear, and points of light often seem to have trails. Aside from distorted vision, its effects on individuals differ. Some feel fatigue in and around their eyes, suffer headaches, and tire quickly when reading. Others complain of poor digestion, dizziness, and irritability.

Middle-age sight (presbyopia)

Sooner or later it comes to us all. As you grow older, your power of accommodation becomes less and less and your ability to focus on near objects becomes impaired. Not only do the ciliary muscles decrease their activity, but more important, your lenses gradually harden so that by about the age of sixty to seventy they're solidified completely and can no longer respond to focusing changes.

You usually notice this impairment of sight around the age of forty-four when the focusing ability of your lenses has decreased by about two-thirds. Women generally notice the condition before men, and so do shorter people.

HOW TO CORRECT OPTICAL PROBLEMS

When you experience any of the above symptoms, visit your optometrist for an examination of your eyes' focusing ability. The use of appropriate lenses placed in front of your eyes can successfully overcome most focal defects by supplementing their internal focusing mechanisms.

You usually have a choice between regular spectacles and contact lenses. Today most contact lenses are made of wafer-thin, splinter-proof plastic and float on a cushion of natural tear fluid to cover only the corneas of your eyes. These microcorneal lenses must be fitted to the contour of your eyes (there are about fifty-six types of eye curve) for comfort and to assure they stay securely in place as you move your eyes.

Lenses have the advantage over spectacles in being cleaned automatically by your eyelids, are seldom dislodged during strenuous activity and sports, and can't shatter by a chance blow. Unfortunately, not everyone can wear them because of eye irritation, allergies, and similar reasons of incompatibility. Your occulist or optometrist will decide with you whether contact lenses or spectacles represent the best way to correct your focal problems. He'll also advise you how best to build up your tolerance to wearing contact lenses. Most men can usually wear them in comfort almost all day after a three-to-four-week break-in period. Tinted contact lenses can change or intensify your natural eye color or disguise defects. Some actors use them to achieve their startling and hypnotic on-screen stares.

Like spectacles, contact lenses can correct short- and longsightedness, astigmatism, and come in bifocal form to help middle-aged sight problems, although the latter is not very practical. Middle-aged sight usually calls for more complicated lenses, as the efficiency of your focusing machinery decreases. This problem can be handled by using different pairs of spectacles or bifocal or trifocal lenses in a single pair, depending upon the demands of the owners and their occupations.

Select spectacles that not only correct your eye problem but make you more handsome

Too many men take the wrong attitude toward wearing glasses. They're embarrassed for vague or imagined reasons like:

"Wearing spectacles means others will know I've an eye defect." So what—almost everyone has or will have some kind of eye defect.

"I won't look virile." Quite true if you select small pink frames inset with rhinestones.

"They detract from my good looks." Seldom if you wear the right style and color frames.

Girls most certainly make passes at fellows with glasses. Spectacles can be very flattering and, in some cases, a godsend. I'm sure you know men who look a hell of a lot better in glasses than without glasses.

Glasses can also be a distinct advantage in business. Some styles will give you a more serious and mature look, and in the hands of an expert, can command attention at meetings. One real advertising pro would remove his spectacles with purposeful movements to attract everyone's attention as soon as he began speaking. He would use them as a pointer to emphasize his remarks, and if he had nothing of any real importance to say, he'd still keep his audience enthralled by folding and unfolding his spectacles (they had five hinges and seemed to shrink to the size of a silver dollar) until he thought up a winning argument.

When selecting your spectacles, give time and thought to finding the frame whose shape, material, and color really do something for your face, not just sit there in front of it. Handmade frames come in forty thousand different combinations of shape, color, and size. You can't tell me that some of them aren't going to make you look better than others. Consider the following when choosing the most flattering frames for your face:

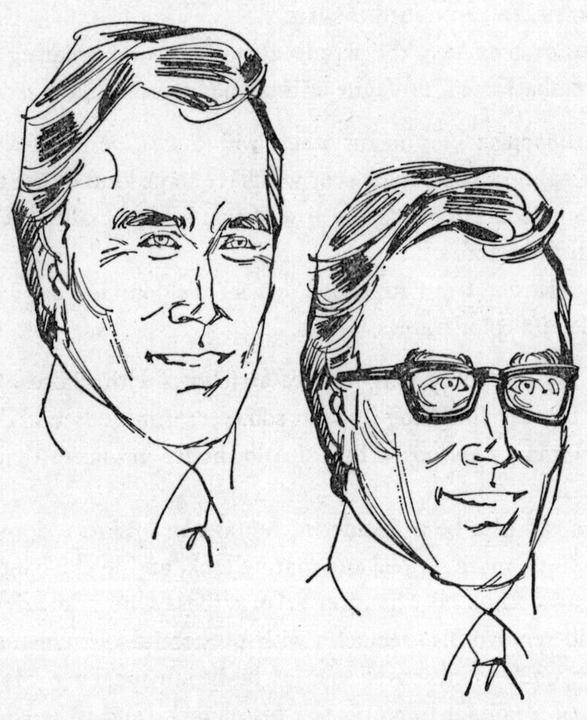

Eyes too close: Compensate with frames greater in depth at their outer ends than at the middle. (See above).

Eyes set far apart: Make them appear closer together with frames greater in depth at the inner end than at the middle.

Excessively angular face: Counterbalance it with a frame emphasizing the curved lines of your face.

Round face: Slim it with frames having pronounced vertical depth.

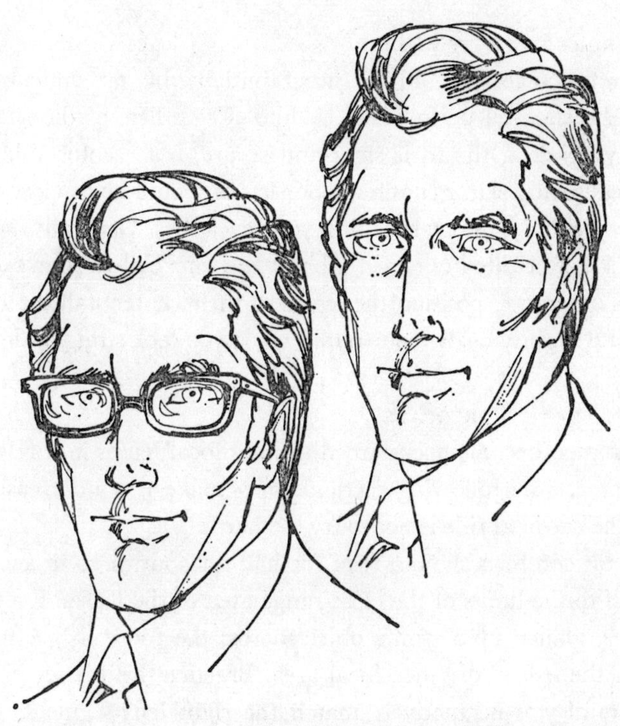

Very long face: Round with frames noticeably more horizontal than vertical, particularly those with flat top and bottom rims.

Long nose: Shrink it with a low-fitting bridge.

Small, turned-up nose: Lengthen with a narrow high-fitting bridge.

Pointed chin: Avoid frames with pointed bottom edges.

Round chin: Avoid rounded lower rims.

Darker-colored frames usually go well with dark hair, lighter colors with fair skin and light hair.

Make sure the frames go well with the shape and thickness of your eyebrows.

Make sure they fit well

Your spectacles should be fitted initially by an optician and should be checked periodically by him. Regardless of the shape of frame you select, the fit is snug and secure, but comfortable, so it won't cause any skin irritation. Your lenses should be as close to the eyes as possible without touching your eyelashes. Generally, spectacles look better tilted outward a bit at the top. Unless your optician decides otherwise, position the lenses so their centers fall directly in front and slightly below your pupils when you look straight ahead.

How to break in bifocals

Most men become accustomed to multifocal lenses in a relatively short time. The following methods may make it a little easier for you. The cardinal rule is not to try too hard.

1. Sit comfortably and read for half an hour or so to accustom yourself to the limits of the close-range area of the lenses. Every few minutes, glance up at some object across the room to get used to finding the lenses' distance focal area. Practice this for several evenings until you instinctively match the right lens segments to the various distances.

2. For the next week or so, wear your bifocals while walking around your home, office, or other familiar place. Start with an hour a day and, as you feel more comfortable with your bifocals, add an hour each day until you're up to about eight hours.

3. Follow the same procedure in less familiar or strange locations. After this has been completed, you should be comfortable and at home with your bifocals under any conditions.

Proper care of your spectacles is essential

Wash your spectacles once a day in warm, soapy water, special cleaning fluids, or even use cologne, or wine to remove oil and dirt. While washing and polishing, hold only the rims surrounding the lenses, never the bridge, hinges, or earpieces. Don't breathe on the lenses or polish them while dry.

When you put on or take off your spectacles, always grasp them at the hinges, put them face up on a safe surface or place them face down in their case when not in use. This treatment should keep your frames from bending out of shape and the lenses free from scratches and pits.

How to stop your lenses from misting in winter

Winter athletes can stop their lenses from misting by lightly smearing a bit of dry soap over them and polishing. The remaining thin film of oil should control misting all day.

PROTECT YOUR EYES FROM THE SUN

High intensities of ultraviolet, infrared, and even visible light can tire your eyes and cause a great deal of damage. These intensities can occur at high altitudes when looking near the sun, when sunlight reflects off water, sand, snow, or smooth bright surfaces, from the mercury vapor or arc lamps in film and TV studios, and the like. If you were to look directly at the sun, your cornea and lens would act like magnifying glasses to literally burn out your fovea centralis so you could not focus sharply on anything ever again. Rather than go into all the variations of occupational protective spectacles, only the common sunglasses, which we all wear at one time or another, will be covered.

WHICH ARE THE BEST SUNGLASSES?

You want glasses that both filter out harmful infrared and ultraviolet rays *and* reduce glare. Too many men (and women) mistakenly select sunglasses based upon the style of the frames, not the protection given by the lenses. Unfortunately, the ability of tinted glass and plastic lenses to filter out and control the visible and invisible rays of the sun differs widely. Some may lull you into a false sense of security while offering relatively little eye protection. Price isn't necessarily an indication of lens quality. In a recent survey the most expensive pair of sunglasses tested turned out to be the worst buy.

The wisest thing to do is ask your oculist or a qualified optician to recommend the brand of lenses that best filter out harmful rays and glare. Then look until you find them.

It's difficult to generalize in this area, but tinted glass lenses made by reputable firms are generally superior in filtering out infrared and ultraviolet rays and pretty good at cutting down on visible light. Polaroid material by itself effectively cuts out reflected glare and transmits low levels of visible light, but it is less successful in filtering out the invisible rays. Therefore, lenses with which the material is combined must compensate for this weakness. Remember, all Polaroid glasses are not the same.

If you're going to subject sunglasses to rough use, get lenses of reinforced or toughened glass or those with a thin interlayer of plastic. They stand greater impact than ordinary lens glass and won't shatter into sharp splinters.

Obviously, have sunglasses fitted like proper spectacles so they're comfortable, secure, and don't interfere with your vision.

WHEN NOT TO WEAR SUNGLASSES

Wear dark glasses only when light conditions make their use necessary. Don't become addicted to them. Unless otherwise recommended by your doctor or oculist, they shouldn't be worn on dull days, after sunset, or indoors no matter how glamorous you think you look. Making a habit of this can cause your eyes to become extrasensitive to infrared and ultraviolet rays as well as normal bright sunlight. These effects are temporary (lasting up to a month) but can cause you unnecessary distress.

Don't wear sunglasses while driving at night to ease the oncoming dazzle of headlights. They don't really cut down the glare, and they dangerously impair the night vision you need to sort out other potential road problems.

STAY ALERT TO THE SYMPTOMS OF EYE DISEASE AND OTHER PROBLEMS

Aside from the more innocent optical difficulties discussed earlier, there are other problems that can harm your eyes and, if not treated in time, may result in impaired vision or blindness. Keep alert for these symptoms and, should they occur, consult an oculist (ophthalmologist), who is a medical doctor trained to diagnose and treat (surgically if necessary) these problems.

FIRST, WHAT NOT TO WORRY ABOUT

Before going further, let's get rid of a few of the common myths concerning the causes and treatment of eye problems. First of all, no permanent damage comes from eyestrain, incorrect spectacles or lack of spectacles when you need them. Close work won't aggravate myopia.

Don't worry about TV. Excessive viewing doesn't hurt your eyes, nor does it matter if other lights in the room are on or off, except for your own comfort. You should, however, make sure your TV picture is steady and free from distortion and look up from time to time to rest your eyes.

Carrots won't improve your vision in the dark because you get more than enough vitamin A for your eyes' needs from a normal balanced diet. Eye exercises won't improve a long- or shortsighted condition because the problems usually depend on the size and shape of your eyes, not with their muscles.

Finally, there's no truth to the often heard statement that eyes of one color are stronger than those of another. A single pigment is responsible for the entire wide range of eye colors. The more of this pigment in your irises, the darker your eyes. Lesser amounts give pale blue and light gray colors. If irises totally lack pigment, the underlying blood vessels show through, resulting in pink, albino eyes.

The squint (heterotropia)

Six pairs of tiny muscles control the movement of your eyes. During the first years of life, a complex conditioned response of these muscles keeps most babies' eyes correctly synchronized. While a child matures, this reflex becomes consolidated as his brain builds up a relationship between the accommodation needed to focus both eyes and the muscle action which causes them to converge as an object moves closer. He thus learns that only by keeping his eyes parallel can he integrate the image formed on both retinas into a single three-dimensional image.

If one or more ocular muscles fail to function correctly, you lose the co-ordination movement of your eyes. Only one eye looks directly at an object, the other off to its side. In severe cases where eye alignment cannot be maintained, the brain relies basically on the information received from only the good eye, ignoring the blurred and confusing information from the deviated one. Scientifically this condition is called a squint. You've commonly heard it referred to as cross-eyes, walleyes, etc. It may be inherited, develop gradually in childhood because of optical deviation between your eyes, or occur suddenly at any time.

Almost all of us have some degree of squint which we instinctively fight in order to keep our three-dimensional vision. The actual deviation of someone's eyes may not be noticeable until after he's done a lot of close work or lets his guard down when sleepy or exhausted and, sometimes, when drunk. You may have watched this phenomenon happen in some of your friends late on a boozy evening. The constant muscle effort needed to maintain proper eye alignment may give you headaches and pain around your eyes, a temporary blurring of vision, or a feeling of nausea or vertigo. You can usually get some temporary relief by closing one eye. Squint can be cured occasionally in children under seven years by covering the dominant eye to force the deviated one to regain is lost vision, and by using spectacles. After this age the muscle of the eye becomes hyperdeveloped, and muscle surgery is usually necessary to realign the eyes. In addition, spectacles are usually needed to correct the optical problems.

Cataracts

A cataract affects vision by interfering with the transparency of your lens and so obstructs the passage of light waves moving through to the retina. The lens becomes opaque or clouded in spots which slowly grow for years until perception of even the largest object can be lost.

You usually notice the first symptoms of a cataract when your vision becomes slightly misty and/or spots appear before your eyes. Often the afflicted eye picks up more than one image of objects, particularly small, bright ones. In old age, cataracts can also affect color perception of blues, violets, and sometimes yellow. The later works of Renoir and Turner reflect this color distortion.

Cataracts most commonly affect old eyes. Almost everyone over the age of seventy has a few small ones, but fortunately they grow so slowly that their vision usually isn't seriously impaired during their lifetime.

Occasionally cataracts are present at birth or develop in early childhood as the lens grows. In these cases the opaque areas usually remain about the same throughout life.

Currently no treatment has been found to arrest cataract growth. In severe cases the opaque lens is removed surgically, after which contact lenses or spectacles are worn to compensate for the lost focusing power of the lens.

GLAUCOMA

One or two people in every hundred over the age of forty will contract this condition, which causes about a third of all blindness in later life. Glaucoma hits women more than men and tends to affect longsighted people and those who are anxious and under tension. It usually seems hereditary, but can be brought on by a previous inflammatory eye disease or physical injury.

Glaucoma is a buildup of pressure in your eyes caused by an imbalance between the rate of production of aqueous humor and the rate at which this liquid drains out of the eye. In about 10 per cent of the cases, the imbalance is caused by a complete blockage of the drainage canals. Unable to escape, the aqueous humor builds up considerable pressure and creates intense pain radiating from your eyes and reduces your vision. The attack may have been preceded by several years of frequent and short attacks of cloudy or misty vision and often a decline in your power of accommodation which necessitated frequent changes in the power of your reading glasses. In most of these cases, a small operation may be used to surgically improve the drainage. It results in a permanent cure.

Unfortunately, in 90 per cent of the cases of glaucoma, there are no really noticeable symptoms, and the condition isn't recognized until after considerable visual loss. In these cases, the drainage canals become partially blocked so only a small (but damaging) increase in pressure builds up to force out the aqueous humor. As glaucoma becomes relatively advanced, you begin to lose your peripheral vision and night vision. Night driving becomes more difficult, and you're more likely to stumble in the dark. The other warning sign is having to change the prescription of your glasses more frequently than normal. (After the age of forty-three, you should expect to change your prescription only every two to three years.) This form of glaucoma is usually treated medically with drugs to open the drainage canals. The treatment must be carried on for the rest of your life.

Conjunctivitis

The thin conjunctiva, which protects your cornea, contains very few tiny blood vessels which, when inflamed, give you the common bloodshot eye. Conjunctivitis is characterized by this inflammation and also a sticky discharge. Bacterial or viral infection usually causes it, but allergies or nervous disease may also be responsible. Various lotions and ointments can soothe the conjunctiva, but the quickest cure lies with antibiotics.

Blepharitis

Blepharitis, in which inflammation occurs at the roots of your eyelashes, may arise if you've a tendency to dry skin, dandruff, or acne. It may also be caused through an allergic reaction to substances trapped around the eyelashes. Actors sometimes develop this inflammation because of mild allergy to some types of makeup. If you fall into this category, be sure to keep this area clean.

Color blindness

Only rarely do men find themselves totally color-blind, seeing only shades of white, black, and gray. Others suffer varying degrees of color blindness, some seeing red and green as gray, some yellow and blue as gray, and some seeing colors less bright than normal.

Men suffer more from this condition than women. We know little of its causes, although it's often transmitted by heredity from an unafflicted mother to her male offspring. There's no known cure.

A SUMMARY OF THE CARE FOR YOUR EYES AND SIGHT

Follow these rules to care for eyes and protect your sight:

1. Have your eyes examined every few years (or more often if necessary) for focal problems by an optometrist or oculist, particularly if you're over forty.

2. Seek immediate help from an ophthalmologist if you encounter any of the following symptoms:

- a squint
- misty or spotty vision
- eyestrain, headaches, and eye fatigue
- inflammation of your eyes or eyelids accompanied by a sticky discharge
- temporary loss of sight for any reason
- an injury such as a knock causing a black eye or any infection of the eye
- frequent need to change the lenses in your spectacles

3. Wear spectacles or contact lenses to correct focus defects and ease eyestrain. Have their fit checked periodically by an optician.

4. Protect your eyes from high intensities of sunlight and artificial illumination with effective sunglasses or special occupational work glasses. Where danger exists, also protect them from flying particles with safety glasses. If your regular spectacles or sunglasses get rough treatment, make sure they're made of hardened or shatter-proof glass. Wear contact lenses for sports if you can.

5. Don't overwear your sunglasses—only when light conditions call for them.

6. Carefully remove any irritating particle that gets into your eye; *never* rub it. Wash your eye with clean water or a mild salt

solution or pull back the eyelids and gently remove the particle with the dampened (not with saliva) corner of a clean handkerchief. If the particle doesn't come out within a few minutes, cover your eye with soft cloth or gauze and go at once to your nearest oculist, optometrist, or hospital for treatment.

7. Under normal conditions bathing the eyes of older children and adults isn't necessary, as your natural tear fluid cleans and soothes them for you. Use cosmetic eye lotions which contract the blood vessels in the conjunctiva only when necessary for important appearance, and not too frequently.

8. Make sure you have plenty of light when using your eyes for close work like reading, writing, and fly winding. If not, you'll tire your eyes more quickly. Also work under indirect or diffused light.

9. When watching TV, make sure you tune the set well to eliminate unsteady and distorted pictures which can cause eye-strain. Don't fix your stare on the tube. Glance about the room from time to time to change the focus of your eyes, which helps relax them.

CHAPTER 7

Teeth: An Attractive Smile Wins Friends and Influences People

When you give a warm, welcoming smile to a new business contact, does he think to himself, "What a nice fellow; I'd like to know him better," or "Gosh, look at those teeth!"? For years I've been mystified by one of the most fastidiously dressed and groomed men in the "international" set who appears oblivious to the fact that every time he opens his mouth he destroys his beautifully constructed image. All elegance evaporates when eyes rivet on several discolored and crooked teeth smack in the center of his smile. I'm not the only one who's wondered why he hasn't diverted the price of a few of his custom-tailored suits to a good dentist.

You certainly know how important a good smile is to the success of your appearance and personality, and you have no excuse for not having a really great one, no matter how nature may have started you off. All you have to know is how to give your teeth and gums the right care and how to take advantage of the various dental skills available to you today.

Instead of this, look what most men inflict upon themselves because they just don't take good enough care of their teeth. Riddled with caries (cavities) when young, as we move into middle age more than half of us can expect gum problems (periodontal disease) which may lead to losing our teeth. A United States Army survey indicated that every one hundred inductees required about 600 fillings, 112 extractions, 40 bridges, 21 crowns, 18 partial dentures, and 1 full denture. It has been estimated that the cost of repairing all the damage caused just by caries in the United States would run about ten billion dollars each year. Compare that to the national debt.

In Britain the problem appears even worse because of dietary habits and the lack of awareness of the need for preventative dental treatment. While the average American uses about eight standard tubes of toothpaste each year, the average Briton uses only three. A third of all British adults have no natural teeth and wear full dentures. Don't think that figure applies only to the poor; 30 per cent of those in high social groups have no natural teeth.

In contrast to this dental devastation, my dentist promised that if I'd co-operate with him, I'd keep every tooth in my head looking good for life. How about you?

THE IDEAL SET OF TEETH

There can be no single set of standards for the "ideal" color and shape of teeth, because they must fit each person's inherited coloring and the shape of his face. We do have standards, however, for the ideal cleanliness, alignment, and condition of teeth and gums.

Color: The color of your teeth should harmonize naturally with your skin and hair color. Teeth should be light, but not pure white. Of greatest importance, they should be free of stains and discoloration.

Shape: Their shape (square, round, or rectangular) fits well with the shape of your face, and the size of each tooth should be in proportion to the others.

Cleanliness: Clean teeth have no external stains, film of plaque, and no deposits of calculus (tartar).

Alignment: Your teeth shouldn't be overcrowded or crooked, but evenly spaced without obvious gaps. Their tips form an even line consistent with a good matched bite between your upper and lower jaws.

Condition: Ideal teeth have no caries, but those that do exist should be well filled and not noticeable when you smile or talk. Any crowns or replacement teeth will be indistinguishable from your natural ones in color and shape.

Gums: Gums are firm, pink, and *clean,* pressing against the tooth enamel to protect the sensitive and vulnerable neck of your teeth.

HOW TO KEEP YOUR TEETH . . . AND KEEP THEM LOOKING GOOD

Evolution hasn't finished with your teeth yet. Two to three thousand years ago, men had between thirty-six and forty teeth to tear and grind their food. Today one normally has thirty-two teeth. It's predicted men will only have twenty in another few thousand years, but you'd better count on looking after all thirty-two of yours for quite a while.

Proper tooth care has four basic objectives: keeping teeth strong, inhibiting tooth decay, stopping gum disease, and preserving the natural whiteness of your teeth.

Keeping your teeth strong

Each of your teeth has four parts with differing degrees of sensitivity and hardness: the hard **enamel** of the exposed cutting and grinding surfaces; the more fragile and sensitive **dentine**; the very sensitive **pulp** which contains blood vessel and nerves; and the hard **cementum** layer protecting the root and neck of your tooth. The **alveolar ligaments** hold your teeth firmly in their sockets in your jawbone.

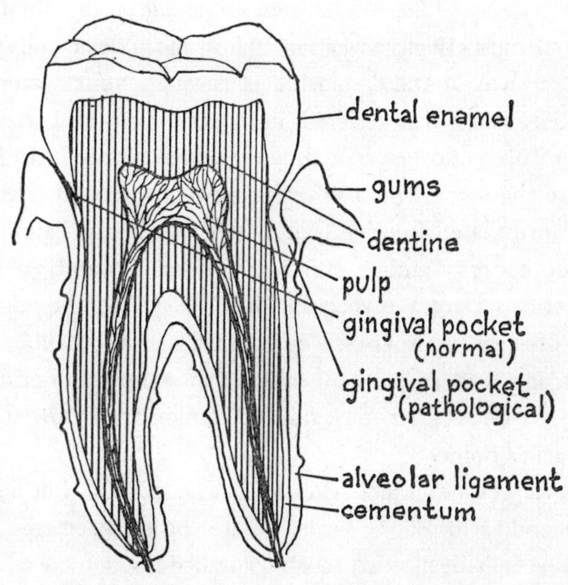

You have no control over the inherited strength of your teeth, but you certainly do over your general health and diet, both of which affect not only the strength of your teeth but the condition of your gums.

Eat the right foods. Hard and fibrous foods, which need chewing, massage your gums and promote good circulation of blood to the gingival areas. Through friction they also help clean some plaque from your teeth and increase the flow of saliva to wash away food particles. Fruit, vegetables, and dairy and animal foods contain the vitamins C and D and calcium essential to strong teeth and healthy gums. (See Chapter 10.)

Use fluoride. During the formative years from womb up to six, fluoride interacts with tooth enamel to form a stronger compound which is more resistant to acid attack. In the following years, fluoride continues to give tooth protection, but the experts don't really know why. Thus aside from brushing, using fluoride represents your most effective weapon against tooth decay today.

The best way to take fluoride is through your water supply. Fluoridated water has resulted in a reduction of caries among children of up to 60 per cent. If your water supply lacks fluorides, tablets are the second most effective way of taking it. Next comes properly formulated fluoride toothpastes which can be expected to reduce tooth decay among children between 20 and 30 per cent. The American Dental Association has recognized the effectiveness of many of these toothpastes. Your dentist can also paint your teeth with a strong 8 to 10 per cent solution of stannous fluoride several times a year or may recommend and demonstrate how to apply a fluoride gel at home.

Can you get too much fluoride? Too high a fluoride intake during a child's formative years, before the teeth emerge from his gums, can result in mottled tooth color. Adults don't seem affected by overdoses in this way. Properly fluoridated water in conjunction with a fluoride toothpaste shouldn't have any adverse effects on adults' or children's teeth.

Various countries have devised ways of making sure their people get enough fluoride. The Dutch put it in bread and the Swiss in salt. Some manufacturers experiment from time to time with adding fluoride to candy, but this seems to me rather like putting penicillin around a bullet.

Inhibiting tooth decay

You can attribute most of the disease and decay in your mouth to one thing, **plaque.** Plaque starts forming within hours of brushing. First, protein from saliva creates a tenacious film over your teeth. A second layer of bacterial enzymes in your mouth sticks to this base. Food debris forms the third layer. Technically only the second layer is plaque, but for simplicity sake I'll refer to all three as plaque. It can vary from a transparent film to a soft yellow-white layer of considerable thickness.

The bacteria immediately attack the food particles trapped next to them and make acids which the plaque holds firmly against your tooth enamel and exposed dentine. Thus within moments of eating or drinking, the decay process in your mouth begins.

Research is under way to find agents that will inhibit the decay process. A group of hospital patients under prolonged treatment with penicillin experienced a significant reduction in tooth decay. Apparently this drug affected the harmful bacteria in their mouths. Adding antibacterial agents, like penicillin, to toothpaste may be possible one day, but to my knowledge no leading dentifrice now contains an effective antibiotic. Manufacturers also search for dentifrice additives to inhibit the acid-making process between mouth bacteria and food. To date claims that these additives will protect teeth against caries haven't been substantiated to the satisfaction of dental authorities.

Cut down on sweet foods that harm your teeth. Evidence shows an indisputable link between tooth decay and carbohydrates, particularly sugar. (Fats and protein appear relatively innocent.) Within the carbohydrate family, sugars are more harmful than starches, but the latter do their share of damage. If you doubt that starchy carbohydrates like bread have a high sugar content, simply hold a piece of white bread in your mouth for a minute or two. You'll taste its sweetness.

Refined sugar (sucrose) appears the worst offender, and yet the average Briton consumes about two pounds of it every week. Sticky toffee, jellies, cakes, and other high-sugar foods and drinks literally dissolve your teeth away. During sugar rationing in World War II, the caries rate among British children dropped dramatically.

Stop between-meal snacks. Every time you eat, no matter how little, you're laying down another layer of food debris to be turned into tooth-dissolving acids. Try to stick to three basic meals a day. If you must have snacks in between, use saccharin in your coffee or tea, forget sweet things, and nibble vegetables and cheese instead. End every meal or snack with a nonsugar drink to help wash down food particles left in your mouth.

Keep your teeth clean. There's no doubt about it, the most effective way to inhibit tooth decay is to clean away the film of plaque covering your teeth, and the best way to do that is with the old-fashioned toothbrush and toothpaste. The more often you brush away plaque, the more effective your fight against tooth decay. I'll cover the most effective brushing technique later in this chapter.

Stopping gum (periodontal) disease

The older you get, the less trouble you'll have with caries. Your tooth enamel gets more brittle, and dental work usually consists of replacing existing fillings. But you're not out of the woods yet. Gum disease, rather than caries, represents the major threat to your teeth in middle and later life. And once again, plaque is held responsible for a lot of this periodontal trouble.

Although not very noticeable, gum disease often starts in your late teens and early twenties when your body falls under the various stresses of adolescence and growing up: late nights, nervous tensions, smoking, freaky and unbalanced diets, and the like. Receding gums and allied diseases become more pronounced with age (about thirty-five years) and grow in intensity as your system loses some of its ability to repair itself and fight back. Approximately 15 per cent of you between the ages of twenty and twenty-nine years have exposed tooth root surfaces, while 58 per cent of those in the fifty-to-fifty-nine-year group have exposed roots.

Plaque and the buildup of irritating formations of calculus on your teeth can inflame your gums and encourage gingival pockets to develop between your teeth and gums. These pockets make perfect bases for infection and gradually increase in size allowing the underlying bone to recede and the anchorage of your teeth to give way. Ultimately this condition can lead to inflammation of your tooth sockets (pyorrhea) which generally results in loose teeth and pus accumulation. You may also suffer the side effects of an upset stomach and foul breath. It's not very attractive, but if caught in time you can usually reverse these problem conditions with treatment.

A forty-year-old friend of mine developed a toothache while his faithful old family dentist was on vacation. With some trepidation he visited a new, but highly recommended man. It proved a very fortunate meeting indeed. After taking one look in Darby's mouth, the new dentist bundled him off to a periodontist who worked for six months to save his teeth, over half of which were in danger of coming loose from advanced gum disease. So much for the old family dentist who hadn't kept up with the advances in his profession. Don't let this sort of thing happen to you.

You can best maintain the health of your gums by **keeping them clean** and **stimulating circulation** through brushing. Have your dentist remove accumulations of calculus every six months. Also make sure he keeps a close watch for potential periodontal trouble. Finally, try to remove as much emotional stress from your life as you possibly can.

It may come as a surprise to you, but research conducted over the last few decades shows a correlation between the increasing levels of tension and stress in our society and a rising incidence of dental problems. Many men find an outlet for their tensions by unconsciously clenching and grinding their teeth during the day and while at sleep. These actions not only wear down their teeth, but can contribute directly to gum recession and tooth loss.

If you suffer from this problem, your dentist may give you a transparent plastic cap (like a football mouth guard) to cover your top teeth during the night. This pliable cap cushions forces and also has a tranquilizing side effect like a child sucking his thumb. Some men become so reliant on this "pacifier" that they wear it throughout the day and often refuse to kick the habit. Fortunately, the cap wears out before real addiction sets in, but this strong reaction certainly reflects the insecurity and tensions under which many men find themselves today.

Preserving the whiteness of your teeth

The color of your teeth depends upon the inherited color of the dentine which shows through the transparent tooth enamel. No matter what the ads imply, there's no such thing as pure white teeth. Put a thin piece of white paper over your teeth and see the dazzling, but artificial, effect. Dentists often have trouble with patients who demand almost pure white dentures or crowns only to come screaming back as soon as they look in their mirrors with horror. Resign yourself to the fact that your teeth will yellow a bit with age. It's the natural result of the thickening of secondary dentine.

Your teeth lose their natural whiteness because the plaque which covers them becomes stained and dirty from smoking, tea, wine, and many foods. You whiten them simply by cleaning off this discoloring layer. The cleaner your teeth, the whiter they'll look—but only to a point.

Sometimes chemical whiteners are used which may actually corrode teeth, but these can be potentially harmful. Rely upon your dentist for periodic intensive cleaning.

THE MOST EFFECTIVE WAY TO CLEAN YOUR TEETH AND GUMS

1. Use the right brush

The latest periodontal research conducted in the United States indicates that the most effective brush for cleaning plaque from your teeth and gums and for massaging your gums is one that contains multitufted, very soft, round-headed bristles. Too hard and sharp bristles can abrade your tooth enamel and irritate sensitive gums.

In addition to this standard toothbrush, you may find a single-tufted, stiffer-bristled brush useful to clean hard-to-reach surfaces like those around fixed bridgework.

Electric toothbrushes with the proper bristles and mechanical action appear to clean teeth as effectively as hand brushes. If you're a lazy brusher, they will obviously do a better job for you, but be careful. The ease and pleasant vibrating sensation may tempt you to overuse them and so inflict too much abrasion on your tooth enamel, dentine, and gums. Dentists are divided on the pros and cons of this type of brush.

2. How to brush your teeth

Remember the old song "I wish I could shimmy like my sister Kate"? Well, keep it in mind every time you brush your teeth because the shimmy is the brush movement that has recently been found most effective for cleaning your teeth and gums. It is recommended by the American Academy of Periodontology.

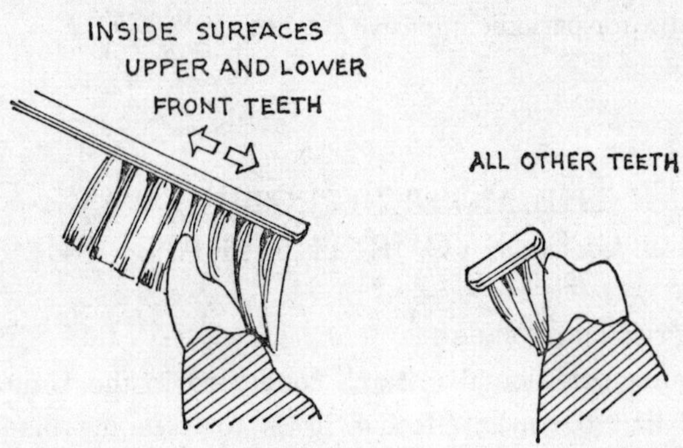

Place your brush at an angle to the junction of your teeth and gums and shimmy it back and forth in horizontal strokes only about the distance of a half a tooth. Do this about six times in front and back of each tooth.

When cleaning the inside surfaces of the upper and lower front incisor teeth, which are difficult to get at, move your brush vertically up and down over your gums and teeth in short gentle strokes.

Over the biting surfaces of your back molar teeth, move the brush back and forth in a scrubbing motion. Next time you visit your dentist, ask him to demonstrate this method for you.

3. Keep the bristles of your brush in good condition

Buy two brushes and alternate them after every use so each has a good chance to dry thoroughly in fresh air. (Don't close them up in toothbrush cases.) From an economy standpoint, two brushes used alternately will last far longer than if used consecutively.

Synthetic bristles are less resilient than natural ones and can be softened by heat, so never subject them to hot water. Always squeeze the tufts of your brush together after every use so they'll dry in their proper shape and thus keep their shape for a longer time.

4. TEST YOUR BRUSHING EFFECTIVENESS

Try the stain test to see how well you're cleaning your teeth. Suck a stain-disclosing tablet (available from pharmacists) which colors plaque red, making it clearly visible on your teeth. After brushing, you'll be able to see the plaque-covered areas that you've missed and that will need more attention in the future.

5. USE THE RIGHT DENTIFRICE FOR YOUR TEETH

Toothpaste has two functions: to clean stains and plaque from your teeth and gums and to freshen your mouth. It normally contains **abrasives,** to physically scrape off plaque; **polishing agents,** to buff your teeth; **humectants,** to resist metabolism of oral bacteria; **foaming agents,** to suspend loosened plaque and debris for easy rinsing; **flavoring** and sweeteners (saccharin type) for a pleasant taste; and **thinners,** which determine the dentifrice's form—powder, paste, or liquid. Some dentifrices also contain additives that act as decay preventatives (fluoride), dull tooth sensitivity, or get rid of particularly difficult stains.

How much abrasive do your teeth need? The cleaning or "whitening" power of a dentifrice depends upon the type and size of the abrasive particles in its formulation. Your need for a harsh or gentle abrasive depends upon how stained your teeth get. For example, smokers' toothpastes usually have harsher abrasive formulas to remove tenacious nicotine stains from teeth. Experiment a bit and decide, with your dentist's help, which brand best suits your needs (this may mean a different brand for different members of your family). Make sure you use enough toothpaste to supply adequate abrasive to all your tooth surfaces. A worm running the full length of the bristle surface should do it. Most of us scrimp.

Tooth desensitizers can take the pain out of brushings. Some of you may suffer particularly sensitive teeth because your dentine has become exposed by gum recession or because of the erosion of protective cementum. Try a dentifrice with an added protein precipitant which forms an artificial barrier to plug the dentine and make its surface insensitive.

In passing, no matter what your great-grandmother told you, table salt isn't a good dentifrice. If used constantly, your teeth will lack luster and become dingy.

6. Use dental floss

After brushing, particularly at night, you should use dental floss to clean food particles and plaque from between your teeth. Draw the floss (either waxed or nonwaxed) gently up and down your tooth surfaces until they feel "squeaky" clean. If the tips of two teeth press together, use a sawing back-and-forth motion, working the floss from the tip down so it lightly touches your gum. This sawing movement dissipates the main force horizontally, not vertically down to slap against and injure delicate gums. When using floss, make sure not to irritate your gums or make them bleed by cutting into them.

7. Rinse thoroughly

Of course it's obvious, but most people don't rinse well. Rinse your mouth thoroughly with plenty of water and/or a mild antiseptic mouthwash to get rid of all the plaque and other debris you've loosened with your brush. It's silly to make the effort to brush your teeth well and then leave half the muck behind to re-collect and start working on your teeth and gums again.

8. Have your teeth "scaled" every six months

The calculus deposits which build up between your teeth and gums should be removed every six months by your dentist. He can remove it manually by scraping your teeth with a small chisel-like tool or with the new ultrasonic scaling unit. When stroked between your gums and teeth, this electric unit emits ultrasonic vibrations which literally shake the calculus off.

At this time, your dentist should thoroughly examine your teeth. It's imperative that he X-ray them to uncover possible root problems below the gum line or detect hidden decay areas between your teeth and around old fillings. Look upon "preventative" dentistry as essential to the long-range health and attractiveness of your teeth and gums.

9. Optional cleaning methods

Wood points and rubber tips: Sufferers of periodontal disease often insert small wooden wedges, triangular in cross section, or rubber tips like those found on some toothbrushes between their teeth to clean them and massage their gums. *Use these points and tips only upon the advice and demonstration of your dentist.* Misuse can be harmful.

The water spray for Buckingham Palace: Rumor has it that during a visit to New York, Prince Philip became so intrigued with the electric water spray unit he found in his hotel bathroom that one was shipped from the States for installation in the Palace.

These machines force pulsating jets of water between and around your teeth at high speed and pressure to remove loose food particles, especially those caught in hard-to-reach places like any permanent bridgework you may have. When using a spray for the first time, set the pressure at low and slowly increase it until you find a comfortable and effective cleaning pressure. Although you may like the sensation at full pressure, it could be too powerful for your gums and help separate them from the teeth. As the water spray doesn't effectively remove plaque, use it in conjunction with the old-fashioned toothbrush. Dentists seldom recommend the water spray during periodontal treatment, and its contribution to over-all oral hygiene is debatable.

HOW COSMETIC AND THERAPEUTIC DENTISTRY CAN IMPROVE YOUR SMILE

Cosmetic dentistry can turn a mediocre or unattractive smile into a real asset. Use it to align uneven and crooked teeth or to replace those that are poorly shaped, chipped, and discolored. Most successful salesmen (and most of us are salesmen in one way or another) depend upon a winning smile. It seems wasteful not to make yours as attractive as possible when dentistry can do it so easily and quickly today.

1. Insist on invisible fillings (restorations) for your teeth

Ask your dentist to fill all highly visible caries in your front and side teeth, particularly those at gum level, with one of the various forms of resin-based ceramics that match your natural tooth color. They're the invisible mending of the dental world. Research on new ranges of dental cements may soon bring translucent preparations that enable your natural tooth color to show through. From a practical standpoint, however, there's no restoration that doesn't discolor a bit sooner or later depending upon your mouth chemistry and diet.

Your dentist will probably use silver amalgams to fill caries in your less visible back teeth. Although more expensive, there's nothing stronger than gold for these bigger fillings. Its durability and nonreaction to saliva and mouth acids make gold the workhorse for bridge and crowns.

2. Cover chipped, discolored, or poorly shaped teeth with crowns

A full crown is usually a cap of gold alloy with an outer layer of porcelain. It's shaped and colored to match your natural tooth (or a more attractive version of it) and telescopes over the old tooth. To fit a crown, the dentist files away much of the offending tooth above the gum line to leave only a peg of dentine extending up from its root. The cap is cemented firmly over this peg. A full crown covers the entire top of your tooth and extends just below your gum line. It's a masterpiece of precision and can seldom be detected from your natural teeth in shape, color, and feel.

Lots of actors and models have had many of their front teeth crowned for absolutely perfect smiles. The man in the photograph section effectively replaced a broken front tooth with a crown. Aside from their good looks, crowns have therapeutic value in replacing part or all of a tooth so decayed or filled with metal that it can't support further repair work.

3. Fill gaps between your teeth and separate overcrowded ones

This work can be done with either braces or bridgework. A Middle Eastern executive had three front teeth so bunched together that the center one began to swivel. After extracting that tooth, the constant pressure of a small brace pulled the other two teeth closer together to fill the gap. In what appeared only a matter of months, all his teeth were evenly spaced and straight. You'd never guess that one was missing.

Conversely, the photograph section shows how effectively braces separated and aligned front teeth so overcrowded that they were beginning to turn sideways. It took just over six months.

A gap created by one or more missing teeth can usually be filled to perfection by a dental bridge. Just like a bridge across a river, your teeth on each side of the gap receive full or partial crowns which act as supports to carry the replicas of the missing teeth which are fastened in between. The entire construction is cemented permanently to the supporting natural side teeth. Removable bridges can also be made.

The life of a bridge or crown depends upon the workmanship of the maker, the type of material used, and the chemistry of your mouth. It also depends on the amount of pressure the artificial teeth receive as well as the degree to which your gums recede with age. A minimum of four to five years can be expected, and some crowns may last a lifetime if all the variables are favorable.

If you're unfortunate enough to have lost so many teeth that bridges can't effectively fill the gaps or if your teeth are in generally bad condition, use full or partial dentures to improve your appearance.

Their fit is essential. Your mouth will adapt to a bad fit which can result in a peculiar jaw movement and twitches as you subconsciously push the denture back into place. I'm sure you've noticed others with this "bite of accommodation" which, if left uncorrected, may affect the muscles of their face. With new technology, dentures can sometimes be fixed permanently to pegs of steel alloy implanted in the jaw, assuming its bone factor is correct. This technique isn't always successful and is generally used only in extreme cases. Remember that your mouth structure and shape gradually change, and so your dentures should be checked for fit at least every two years. It would be far better to take good care of your natural teeth and gums so these problems would never come up.

4. Keep your teeth properly aligned

Your jaws are capable of exerting a crushing force of five hundred pounds. It doesn't take a genius to see why a force of this magnitude can loosen uneven teeth, force them out of position, and throw your entire jaw out of line.

To ensure that the pressure of your bite spreads evenly over as many teeth as possible, your dentist should make frequent adjustments to your teeth by filing down uneven surfaces, particularly after filling caries in a biting surface. Crowns, bridges, and reshaping the tips of your teeth, therefore, have a therapeutic value to the health of your teeth and gums as well as a cosmetic one.

Operations carried out by oral surgeons can correct extremely bad jaw and tooth alignment. In the case of protruding teeth, one tooth on each side of the upper jaw is extracted and L-shaped cuts made in the bone. The whole frontal section, involving about six teeth, can then be moved back and tilted into a more natural position.

Move your lower jaw forward. It not only feels peculiar, but your teeth no longer fit together. You've created what's called the Hapsburg or aggressive jaw, which is of little use to anyone but the bulldog. The problem can be corrected by cutting the lower jaw on both sides and removing two sections of bone. The jaw can then be pushed back into place. Spectacular results are obtained, and it doesn't leave a scar, as the operation can be performed completely from within the mouth.

One last word on the subject of your smile. I don't mean you to go overboard in a completely narcissistic quest for the "perfect" smile. If we all had one, cocktail parties would be dazzling bores. My object has been to point out how obvious dental flaws can detract from your over-all appearance and business effectiveness, and explain how they can be stopped or corrected. Don't be self-conscious about minor flaws which nobody really notices. Keep these, because they tend to give your smile its own distinct and appealing personality.

Chapter 8

Hands: Well-groomed Hands Have Character

Fictional detectives like Agatha Christie's Hercule Poirot rely on the condition of the victim's hands and nails to discover his occupation and social position. Aside from a few other things, beauty experts could tell Monsieur Poirot that this ain't necessarily so. I've seen some pretty bad examples extending from the sleeves of business suits around boardroom tables.

Most men will probably never have perfect, flawless hands, but at least they can keep what they've got attractive and well groomed—and in this case, well groomed doesn't just mean clean. The other two practical criteria for judging your hands are the supple condition of their skin and the attractiveness of the fingernails. The skin should be as youthful-looking as possible, elastic, smooth, soft, and plump—not taut, dry, and cracked. Nails will be discussed in the next chapter.

I've ruled out hand shape as a criterion because it's something over which you have no control. Minor deformities, scars, etc., are to be expected because active men have accidents, and, if anything, these "flaws" add character and individuality to your hands the way a dueling scar does to a cheek.

HOW TO KEEP YOUR HANDS IN GOOD CONDITION

1. PROTECT YOUR HANDS

Constant flexing and exposure to extreme conditions imposed by your work and environment make the skin of your hands one of the first parts of your body to deteriorate and show age. Friction callouses and blisters your skin, physical work can puncture and tear it, and environmental conditions chap and dry it.

Your own common sense and using gloves when practical give your hands their greatest protection. You can get gloves for almost every condition and degree of flexibility that you're likely to encounter in your work and leisure activities. Keep several pairs with your tools and gardening equipment and near at hand so you'll get used to wearing them. If you're going to do really dirty work, wear a thin pair of clean cotton gloves under the heavier working pair to keep out dirt or grease and cut down the friction. Unlike cotton gloves, don't wear rubber ones longer than absolutely necessary because they make your skin perspire and lose its natural oils.

2. CLEAN YOUR HANDS CAREFULLY

When it comes to cleaning, you are your hands' worst enemy. Like most men, you probably plunge them in hot water, rub them with soaps and chemical cleaners, scrub them with metal files. This easy routine has been cleverly designed and passed from father to son to dry and abrade your skin, rob it of protective oils, and age it.

All these actions become even more damaging as your skin matures, becomes thinner, drier, and less elastic.

Proper cleaning should be a gentle and relatively simple procedure which depends on using the right types of products and methods for the degree of dirt and grease you have to remove.

Clean **extremely dirty hands** in two stages. First, massage in a water solution or cream cleaner (plain olive oil is fine for this purpose) to loosen imbedded grime and wipe it away with a tissue. Then wash your hands in the usual way with soap and water.

3. Keep your skin supple

Massage your hands with a cream or lotion containing a natural oil like lanolin at least once a day after washing to replace the skin oils you've removed. Wipe off excess cream with a tissue (or rub your hands over your arms or any other skin that could use a little moisturizing cream; then use the tissue). The film that remains will help your skin retain moisture and protect it from drying. If you have a real dryness problem and haven't planned any nocturnal activity, apply the cream before retiring. The drier your skin, the more often you should use a hand cream during the day. Avoid glycerin or glycerin products which may produce only temporary benefits.

You can make an excellent night cream recommended by the Hand & Nail Culture Institute with ingredients from your local pharmacist.

> Combine: 4 tablespoons lanolin, 4 tablespoons white petroleum, 4 tablespoons cold cream, and 4 tablespoons almond oil. Beat the mixture with a wooden spoon in a bowl immersed in hot water until you get a rich, creamy consistency. Add more almond oil if needed. You can also add a little fragrance. Keep the cream in an airtight jar.

Because of its consistency, this hand cream isn't suitable for daytime use, nor should it be applied on skin if it needs special treatment creams. Your pharmacist can recommend many natural oil hand creams as well as medicated salves for problem conditions.

4. How to remove calluses

If you find them unattractive, remove calluses by gently rubbing them a little each day with the fine side of an emery board. From a realistic standpoint, you can only remove calluses permanently by getting rid of their cause. To change your work or leisure activities for this reason seems a little extreme unless you're an avid narcissist.

5. Get rid of stains

Stains of a onetime nature like ink or iodine will gradually disappear with washing and the natural shedding of skin tissue. If you want the job done faster, use lemon juice, a mild bleach, or a mild stain remover. Here's a simple do-it-yourself stain remover:

> Add 1 tablespoon ammonia and 8 tablespoons pure lemon juice to 8 tablespoons weak peroxide. Don't shake, but stir the mixture. If you keep it in an airtight bottle with an inch of space at the top, it will last some time.

Removing unattractive brown **nicotine stains** from your fingers can be difficult and requires frequent treatment. Rub the stain gently with a pumice stone and then apply some of the stain remover described above or, depending on the severity of the stain, straight weak peroxide. Don't use a strong bleach which might harm your skin. Rather than go to all this bother, have you thought of a cigarette holder?

6. Ease minor burns

Men are always burning their fingers with matches, tools, or, through inexperience, around the stove. When this happens, react instantly by pressing the burn to the lobe of your ear. Your lobe will draw off much of the heat. It's said this prompt action frequently helps reduce the pain and blister. Unless you're a Harry Houdini or want to keep a chiropractor in business, limit the earlobe treatment to your fingers.

7. Do hand exercises

When your hands feel tired or cramped from long periods of writing or some similar activity, revive them with a few exercises.

- Try to touch all your fingertips at once to the point where your fingers join your palms, and then stretch your hands and fingers to their fullest extent. Relax and repeat.
- Shake your hands vigorously from loose wrists so that the fingertips slap each other.

Chapter 9

Fingernails: So You Think You've Got Good Ones?

Next time you take your favorite girl out to dinner, glance down at your hands and nails against the white tablecloth surrounded by silver and crystal. Do the smooth well-shaped surfaces of your nails and cuticles fit this rather elegant and intimate situation, or do they belong out on the prairie next to the old chuck wagon?

Others notice your fingernails more than you suspect. Are they well groomed and shaped? Most men, if pushed, would probably answer yes, and they'd probably be wrong. It's because you get so used to seeing your nails every day that you think they're great as long as they're not dirty. But like hands, cleanliness is only one criterion for good fingernails.

THE PERFECT SET OF NAILS

All your fingernails should grow with complete freedom from the cuticle down to the very tips of your fingers, just as a river flows smoothly along its bed. The nail grooves on each side should be parallel, and smooth folds of skin should envelope your nails almost to their tips. The cuticles look even, not broken or torn, and you should be able to pass the tip of an orange stick under them.

The pink area of each nail should be as large as possible and reach nearly to your fingertips. The white free edges are shaped to harmonize with the contours of the ends of your fingers, not filed to a point or an exaggerated oval—and they're clean. The nails themselves feel strong and flexible, have a bright, clear color and a smooth, lustrous surface.

IT'S EASY TO HAVE NEAR PERFECT FINGERNAILS

Most of us justify the condition of our nails by saying that active men can't possibly expect to have good-looking nails, let alone have perfect ones. This was my reaction until I looked further into the subject and found that the nails of many men around me were noticeably better than mine, and with just a little extra care could have met all the criteria listed above. This woke my competitive spirit and I decided to make the supreme effort, but much to my surprise it was so simple there wasn't really very much effort involved. Depending upon your activities, within two weeks of following this grooming regimen, your cuticles and surrounding skin should look almost perfect. Then it's a matter of letting your nails grow out to their proper length and shaping them.

1. PROTECT YOUR EMBRYO NAILS

Your nail plates grow from embryo nails which lie just beneath your skin in a soft, jelly state. As your nails grow out and harden, they remain attached to beds of soft tissue containing the small blood vessels which supply the embryos with nourishment and give the pink color to your nails. The nail plates are made of protein like that of your hair and skin, and lesser amounts of calcium, phosphorus, and trace metals like arsenic. (That's why Lucretia Borgia and her imitators were reputed to slip ground fingernails into the soup and wine of their intended victims.)

The cuticles surrounding your nails are clear rims of dead skin to protect the living skin and the embryos from infection. Thus nature has done all it can to protect your delicate embryo nails from injury and infection; the rest is up to you. Make sure you, or your manicurist, don't put too much pressure on or dig into this area, and keep your fingers out of car doors and punch presses.

2. SHAPE YOUR NAILS

Start the actual grooming process by working on the shape of your nails. If the free edges don't extend to the very tips of your fingers or run too far down along the sides of your nails, correct this by letting your nails grow out gradually while making sure they stay attached to their beds when cleaning them. Encourage the pink areas to grow out to the sides and almost to the tip of each nail.

It takes the average nail about six months to grow from embryo to tip. (The longest fingernail ever recorded was 22¾ inches and belonged to a Chinese priest. He must have gone for almost four years without cutting it.) Nails grow faster among the young and with increased circulation. That's why right-handed people find the nails of their right hand need trimming more often than those of their left.

File your nail edges smooth and keep them that way so you're not tempted to pick and bite at them. Trim them as little as possible until they grow straight to the tips of your fingers, then shape them to coincide with the curved ends of the fingers. Use a triple-cut metal file or an emery board. Never saw back and forth because this will roughen your nail edge and disturb the nail bed. File in the same direction, from the sides to the center point.

3. Encourage the skin to cover the nail sides

Don't pick at the nail grooves or scrape the sides of your nails when cleaning them. The small pieces of hard skin that form at the sides in the grooves are new nails and should be allowed to remain attached.

Keep your skin grooves from drying and peeling by massaging them and your cuticles with hand cream or oil every day. Always massage in one direction, toward the tip of the finger. Trim away carefully any loose pieces of skin to remove the temptation to pick them.

4. Lift your cuticles

Attractive cuticles are essential to attractive nails. You want to keep them detached from the nail plates so they'll stay smooth and won't tear. If you don't do this as your nails grow, the cuticles will be stretched forward until they break and peel back in the form of ragged edges and hangnails.

You "lift" a cuticle by first softening it in warm water and massaging it with oil. Then gently work the blunt end of a trimmer or hoofstick (see photo section) under your cuticle and pry up the skin with small lifting movements. (In difficult cases you may have to use the blade of your clippers to get under the cuticle for the first time.) Start at a corner and work across the entire cuticle. After freeing it, carefully scrape away the layer of acid deposit on the nail beneath the cuticle; this deposit sticks your cuticle to the nail.

Once lifted, it's easy to keep cuticles free, and you'll start seeing dramatic improvements in their looks. Every few days gently move the tip of an orange stick, trimmer, or hoofstick between your cuticle and nails. The hoofstick was especially designed for this purpose. Slowly rotate its hard rubber, hoof-shaped head back and forth as you move it beneath the cuticles. Remember to keep acid deposits scraped away as they build up.

Warning: Don't push your cuticles back. Some people do it in an attempt to show more of their half-moons. Contrary to popular belief, this damages the cuticles. It stretches and splits them, causing hangnails and possible inflammation.

5. TRIMMING YOUR CUTICLES

Cut cuticles only when necessary. Sometimes when you lift a cuticle for the first time, it's too wide or too thick and hard. For appearance sake, you should cut it back, but cut it very carefully. If too wide, trim away about *half* the skin, leaving a very visible and even rim of clear skin. You may have to repeat this operation every week or so until the cuticle gives up and stops growing out. If you cut away too much skin, you'll stimulate rapid regrowth. Use cuticle clippers, rather than scissors, for better control.

Stretch thick cuticles before cutting them. Grasp sections of the cuticle with your clippers or tweezers and pull the skin, bit by bit, toward your fingertip. Do this gently so as not to tear the skin. When you've stretched the entire cuticle about twice its original width, cut it as described above. You may have to repeat this operation also until the newly thinned cuticle stops growing.

If you're uncertain about your ability to do the initial lifting and trimming, have it done by a well-trained manicurist. She'll demonstrate how to trim the cuticles and keep them free from your nails. (By the way, many manicurists are hacks who do more harm than good. Before you let one touch your nails, ask where she was trained and if she has a degree. After all, you're paying, so demand the best.)

6. GET RID OF HANGNAILS

Hangnails are those little triangles of skin that peel back from beside your nails. They are usually caused by poor grooming, skin dried by detergents, and gardening and similar work as well as nail biting. Don't try to tear them off: this only makes them bigger and deeper. Snip them off as close to the skin as possible with a sharp pair of clippers (see photo section). If serious, cover them with a strip of porous tape until your skin heals. Hangnails represent one of the most irresistible stimuli for nail biting known to man, so get rid of them fast.

7. Cleaning your nails

Here's where a lot of men go wrong, and here's where the basic secret of good grooming lies. Cleaning nails shouldn't be the casual job most of us make of it. If you really want attractive nails, you've got to clean them gently and carefully.

A shadowy gray line divides the pink of your nail bed from the white free edge. Don't mistake this dividing line for dirt and go after it with your cleaning tools. No matter how you dig and push it, the line will be there and all you'll have succeeded in doing is to separate more of your nail from its bed. If you regard this dividing line as an untouchable outer boundary when cleaning, you'll see that it gradually moves forward with nail growth to cut down the size of the dirt-catching free edge. Behind it, the pink area will grow in size.

First a few don'ts. *Don't* use a nail brush if you can possibly avoid it. The sawing action of the stiff bristles separates your nail from its bed, gradually shrinking the pink area. If you must, use a special nail brush and make sure the single row of bristles is at right angles to the under side of your nail so it cleans the nail, not abrades the nail bed. *Don't* use a file. Its sharp edges scratch the underside of your nails, making it easier for them to trap dirt. The file also makes it much too easy to violate the dividing line and so separate your nail from its nail bed.

Now that you've lost your two most favorite cleaning tools, what do you do? Remove limited amounts of dirt from under the free edge with soap and water and a cup-shaped natural sponge (see photo section). Hold the sponge in the palm of your hand with your fingers deep in the hole, which has been well soaped. Open and close your fist. When squeezed, the pressure forces soapy water under the free edge: when released, suction draws out the water and dirt. Continue the flexing action as long as necessary.

To clean out more substantial, imbedded dirt, gently wipe the underside of your free edge with the tip of an orange stick covered by a thin piece of cotton, to which you've applied a little cream or oil (see photo section). The oil will loosen the dirt and the cotton will safely carry it away. (If your hands are still wet from washing or some cream is left under the nails from massaging, you probably won't need to apply extra cream or oil to the cotton.) This cleaning method won't harm the underside of your nail and leaves the dividing line untouched—unless you go mad. If necessary, clean your nail grooves with an orange stick and cotton as well. Keep an orange stick, some cotton, and cream at your office for use when needed during the day.

The less often you have to clean your nails and the less dirt you have to remove, the better. Before undertaking really dirty jobs, pack water-soluble cream under your nails and wear a double pair of gloves. Any dirt that manages to penetrate both gloves won't be able to imbed itself under the nails, and cleaning them will be an easy matter for you.

8. Removing ridges in your nails

Long ridges running the length of your nails usually appear and thicken with age. Overly thick ridges may mar your nails' attractiveness and can be removed by carefully filing them with the fine side of an emery board. Do this about once a month. Filing dulls the nail plate, but a brisk buffing will restore its luster. Don't go too far and file away too much of your nail surface or you'll end with fragile, breakable nails.

9. Buff your nails as the last step in good grooming

Buff your nails briskly to give them a healthy-looking luster and increase circulation in the nail bed. A buffer is simply a piece of chamois stretched over a narrow, pliable base. Always buff in one direction at a time, from the side of your finger to the center of the nail. This encourages the side skin to envelop the nail. Buff at least twelve times from right to left and twelve times in the opposite direction every day, or several times a week.

10. Adding more shine

If you want more shine than you can get from buffing alone, dab a little clear oil on your nails. I recommend against using clear nail enamel which gives the highly artificial shine considered by most circles to be in poor taste for a man.

11. Forget the diet myths

Diet myths abound in this area, but as with hair and skin, most men's diets supply all the nourishment their nails need to stay in good condition. Beauty magazines often blame a lack of calcium for weak nails, but these are the exceptions. There once was a fashion for advising people to consume large quantities of gelatin to strengthen their nails, but there's little proof that this had any positive effect, nor any reason to suppose it would. Many doctors also dispute that high doses of vitamin A and E will strengthen nails, and so I suggest you treat these cures with some skepticism until definitely proved. In short, as long as you have a varied diet, don't worry about your nails.

12. Finally, keep healthy

Your nails act like mirrors to reflect your general health and much of what goes on in your body. Have you noticed that your doctor often checks them for signs of ill health? Heredity and the over-all constitution of your body determine their strength and condition. Anemic people usually have thin brittle nails. A blue tinge indicates poor circulation. Little white dots, aside from being caused by knocks, are said to result from excess acidity in your system due to nervous tension. A severe shock or serious illness often leaves a calling card in the form of a horizontal ridge running across each nail.

A variety of diseases and fungal infections like ringworm, onychia, and paronychia can cause deterioration of the nail plate, discoloration, and inflammation. Because of the seriousness, discomfort, and unattractiveness of many of these conditions, see your doctor at the first sign of trouble.

13. Summary

Combine both the hand and fingernail grooming regimens to cut down time and avoid duplication of effort. Here's how to do it:

1. Clean very dirty hands first with cleansing cream or oil. Wipe with a tissue.

   Wash your hands and nails with soap and water and a cup-shaped sponge.
2. Massage your hands, cuticles, and nail grooves with a hand cream containing a natural oil. Leave some cream under the free edges of the nails.
3. Clean the free edges with an orange stick, cotton, and oil (if needed).
4. Lift cuticles with a hoofstick and scrape away acid deposits beneath if needed.
5. Remove any excess oil or cream from your hands.
6. Trim and file your nails to fit the contours of the fingertips if needed.
7. Trim away any hangnails or rough skin.
8. Buff your nails twelve times in each direction.

CHAPTER 10

Nutrition and Your Health

Not long ago over cocktails, Lady X, looking rather pale and drawn, confided to me that she'd never have to suffer the pain of arthritis; she'd given up eating salt. It seems an older friend of hers had been put on a salt-reduced diet, and, among other things, her arthritis appeared improved.

When I explained that salt was essential to the fluid balance of her body and asked about her doctor's reaction to this self-inflicted scheme, she replied not to worry, that she planned to soak in her bath filled with salt water once every month. Faced with this logic, I retreated from what promised to be a fruitless battle and had another whiskey.

That brief encounter highlights the confusion and the misconceptions with which most people approach nutrition and their diet. They believe in miracle vitamins and foods because they want to believe in them. The food articles that seem to fill every magazine don't really help the confusion. This is unfortunate because nutritional misconceptions can adversely affect your vitality and appearance and be damaging to your health.

This chapter is a purely informative one, designed to clear up the questions you have concerning the effects of your diet on the health and appearance of your body. It will give you the foundation upon which to build better eating habits for better weight control and over-all health.

IS THERE AN IDEAL DIET?

There is an ideal diet, but it varies for each individual. Aside from tasting good, the ideal diet for you supplies the nutrients your body needs for its growth and repair and to keep its other processes functioning correctly. Your food intake must generate sufficient energy to enable your body to perform all its daily activities while holding its weight at a level best suited to your height and build.

Putting together a diet of this type is a lot more simple than you think if you stick to the basic truths, use your common sense, and don't get sidetracked by the latest fads and gobbledygook.

HOW FOODS AFFECT YOUR BODY

You'll probably eat some thirty tons of food in your lifetime (the equivalent of six elephants). Most of that food will have good nutritional value; some will have none.

Food consists of varying combinations of three basic nutrient groups: protein, fats, and carbohydrates. These supply your body with the materials for growth and tissue repair as well as the fuel, or energy, it needs for its daily activity. You measure the energy-giving potential of food in calories.

Food also contains nutrients in the form of minerals and vitamins. These keep your body healthy, aid growth, and help regulate various bodily processes. Although not strictly classified as a nutrient, water is essential to life.

You need protein to repair worn-out tissue

Protein consists of about twenty different amino acids in different combinations. Your body uses these acids to repair worn-out protein in its tissues. It can make about half of the amino acids internally, but depends upon food for the rest.

Animal foods like meat, eggs, milk, cheese, and fish offer you the best and most varied supply of amino acids, but you need protein from other foods as well to get the proper variety and amount of these nutrients.

Why you need minerals

Your body contains many minerals: sodium, chlorine, potassium, calcium (enough lime to whitewash a chicken house), phosphorus, magnesium, fluorine, iron, copper, cobalt, iodine, sulfur, and other trace minerals. The purpose of explaining the function and source of these minerals is to impress you with the importance of eating a wide variety of foods. Men with good, varied diets normally ingest enough of these minerals every day, but if you've got very weird eating habits, you'd better do a rethink.

Sodium, chlorine, and **potassium** help maintain your body's fluid balance. The chief source of sodium and chlorine is salt. Healthy people never have a salt deficiency unless their needs greatly increase due to excessive sweating. Normally we take in ten times more salt than we need and get rid of the excess without any trouble. If, for some reason, you accumulate too much salt in your body, water accumulates with it. Your weight increases and you may develop the condition called dropsy. The most common problems caused by a salt deficiency are dehydration and cramps.

Calcium strengthens your bones and teeth. Nutritionists aren't absolutely sure how much of this mineral you need because various other things in your diet affect the amounts of calcium the body can absorb from food. For example, the outer parts of wheat contain a substance (phytin) that combines with calcium to hinder its absorption. As a result, milled white bread (without phytin) gives your body more calcium than whole wheat bread.

You get high amounts of calcium from milk, cheese, and bread. If you drink a reasonable amount of milk every day, you probably won't run short.

Phosphorus and **magnesium** also help the development and maintenance of good bones and teeth. They're found in most foods.

Fluorine, as we discussed earlier, helps protect your teeth against decay.

Iron fights anemia. It makes the coloring matter (hemoglobin) in your red blood cells. You have enough in your body to make a medium-sized nail. Women need more iron than men because of their regular loss of blood through menstruation.

Although you only need about one two-thousandths of an ounce of iron a day, relatively few foods contain significant amounts. Eggs and meat, particularly liver and organ meats, represent your best source. True to Popeye's claim, spinach contains more iron than any other cooked vegetable.

Copper and **cobalt** work in conjunction with iron to manufacture your red blood cells. You get copper in most nuts and vegetables, and cobalt from vitamin B_{12}. Pernicious anemia strikes if your body can't properly absorb this vitamin.

Iodine plays an important part in controlling the rate at which you use up energy. An enlargement of your thyroid gland can result from a deficiency of this mineral. Fish and other seafoods are your main source of iodine, although in some countries people have to rely upon iodized salt for it.

THE IMPORTANCE OF VITAMINS

Like lubricants to a machine, vitamins keep the working parts of your body going and in good health. Don't look upon them as miracle workers. They're no more important than minerals and protein.

We know of fifteen vitamins, but don't know yet if your body needs them all. Fortunately, most normal diets give you enough vitamins to fill your requirements. Four deserve special attention.

Vitamin A maintains your resistance against disease. It keeps your eyes, skin, and the soft lining of your body tissue from becoming dry and prone to infection. Conversely, a deficiency will lower your resistance to disease and cause dry and rough skin. Eye infections caused by a lack of vitamin A are still common factors in human blindness in several Eastern countries.

You get high levels of vitamin A from milk, butter, and cheese and particularly from the liver of meat and fish, and fish oils. Your body also manufactures it from the carotene found in all green plants and some vegetables like carrots. Therefore, a reasonable diet of dairy foods and green or yellow vegetables will keep you in good supply of this vitamin.

The **B complex vitamins** fight depression and fatigue. A lot of vitamins make up the B complex, and all appear related to your body's metabolism. A deficiency over a period of time will have serious effects. Lack of sufficient **B_1** (thiamine) can cause fatigue, depression, constipation, and indigestion; **riboflavin,** sore, flaking skin, cracked lips, and inflamed eyes; **nicotinamide,** a sore tongue, rough and red skin, along with stomach and mental upset; and **B_{12}**, a type of anemia and degeneration of your nervous system.

Apart from B_{12}, found primarily in animal foods, you can get the other B complex vitamins in varying amounts from most foods. The highest concentration comes from meat, milk, and whole cereals, and particularly in liver, wheat germ, and yeast.

Vitamin C builds up your stamina. A deficiency of this very publicized vitamin causes weakness, loss of stamina and general ill health, faulty teeth development, sore gums, and delayed healing of wounds.

You find it in most fruit and vegetables, especially in oranges, black currants, strawberries, cabbage, and Brussels sprouts. Vitamin C can be lost easily by overcooking or using too much water in cooking.

Vitamin D builds bones. Adult males can manage on very little of this vitamin, but growing children and pregnant women need more of it for the bone-making process. A deficiency of vitamin D can result in rickets.

Most foods contain little or no vitamin D. Some is found in butter and cheese, but the main source lies in animal and fish livers and the oils made from them. Your body also manufactures this vitamin by the action of ultraviolet rays from the sun on your skin. Cats lick their fur, not to clean it, but to get the vitamin D from it.

When are enough vitamins enough?

Hypochondriacs, beware. Extra vitamins don't help; your system gets rid of excess vitamins and minerals. These nutrients circulate through your bloodstream so that every cell can take exactly what it wants for repair and growth. When the cells have satisfied their needs, your body throws off most of the leftovers.

Once your system has all the vitamins it needs, there's nothing that more of any one, or a combination of them, can do for you. Up to the present time it's not been conclusively proved that extra doses of vitamin A or C will stop colds or infection. If your body functions properly and you keep to a varied diet, you'll seldom have to worry about taking special foods or extra vitamins for health. Only infants and expectant or nursing mothers may need some additional nutrients which they can't get from food alone, and I'm sure you don't fall into either of these categories.

Can too many vitamins harm you?

Only rarely can excessive intake of vitamins harm you. Vitamins A and D aren't soluble in water, and so if you take too many of them, they can't be washed out of your blood through your kidneys. Too high a concentration can cause some harm, but this problem is rare and would probably crop up only if you went out of your way to overdose yourself with tablets or fish oils and liver.

How many calories do you need for energy every day?

A calorie is a unit of energy released by your body when it "burns" food. The statement that an ounce of plain chocolate contains 156 calories means that when oxidized in your body tissue, it will release that amount of energy for your body to use in its various activities.

An ounce of chocolate contains 1.6 grams of protein, 10 grams of fats, and 14.9 grams of carbohydrates. Each gram of protein in food can produce about 4 calories; a gram of fat, 9 calories; and a gram of carbohydrate, 4 calories. By simple multiplication you arrive at the 156 calories (or energy) value of the chocolate and can do the same calculation for other foods.

Obviously the number of calories one needs every day varies between individuals and depends upon body size, metabolism, and work load. If you have an average build and metabolism and do an average amount of work, you're likely to burn up about 3,000 calories a day. The average woman uses about 2,500.

At rest, you need approximately eleven basal calories per pound of weight just to maintain your body's basic life processes like breathing and blood circulation. That's almost 2,000 calories if you weigh 180 pounds. You need more calories to stand up, eat, and work. It's estimated that your body requires an additional 25 per cent of your basal calorie level to do light work, 75 per cent more for moderate work, and 100 per cent for hard work. You may need anything from 150 to 200 per cent more to do extremely hard work like digging ditches.

The excess calories from protein, fat, and carbohydrate which your body doesn't need for its maintenance and growth or which it doesn't burn up for energy, are stored as fat. Around 4,000 unburned calories make one pound of fat. Your body won't burn off these fat reserves unless it doesn't get enough energy fuel from its daily food intake. That's what dieting is all about—burning up those reserves.

HOW TO ASSURE YOURSELF A HEALTHY DIET

1. First, fill your nutrient requirements

Your primary objective must be eating those foods that supply the nutrients your body needs for its health and to keep functioning properly. As you've seen, the major sources of vitamins, minerals, and protein differ, and so your diet has to be a varied one.

Two reasonable helpings from each of the following four food groups should give you the main nutrients in pretty nearly the amounts you need every day. A half pint of milk is the daily minimum. If you eat enough milk or cheese, or both, you don't always need foods from Group 1.

Group 1	meat, fish, eggs
Group 2	milk, cheese
Group 3	fruit, vegetables
Group 4	butter, margarine

Group 1 provides you with protein, some B complex vitamins, iron, and some minerals. Milk and cheese have many vitamins, protein, calcium, and some of the other minerals. Group 3 contains vitamins A and C, and Group 4 has vitamins A and D.

2. Then fill your energy requirements

If you eat a simple daily diet composed of only the foods in this four-group formula, you'll have far less than the 3,000 calories needed for energy by the average man. Add more food to this basic diet to meet your particular energy requirements, but do it with discretion and restraint or you'll land yourself with too many calories and an overweight problem. Select foods with high nutritional value and low carbohydrate and calorie content. If you start putting on weight, cut back this added food intake so your body will start burning up fat reserves for energy.

Sugar exemplifies dietary waste. It contains no more than minute traces of vitamins, minerals, and protein and is practically 100 per cent carbohydrate. Even though it has basically no nutritional value, in the wealthier countries the average person consumes about two pounds of sugar a week, accounting for some 3,500 calories. That's the equivalent of depriving your body of nutrients for one day out of every seven and taking on just fuel and probably excess weight.

Beware of fads and faddists who claim miracles. Ask what supposed benefits a particular fad food will give you over and above those you get from your current diet. Honey faddists rave about its vitamins, minerals, and natural sugar which gives you quick energy, but you probably don't need any of these extras. For example, an equal weight of orange juice contains fifty times more vitamin C, and honey can only fill your iron requirements if you eat four or five pounds a day, which is a pretty sickly task. Once absorbed by your body, straight white sugar acts just as effectively as honey to boost energy, and, besides, unless you're a sprinter, you probably don't need honey's fast dose of energy. Your body quite effectively balances sugar levels with energy needed. So if you like honey, eat it, but don't expect miracles.

Before throwing yourself into food fads or crash diets, talk with your doctor. In most cases you'll find you save yourself a lot of trouble and money, and your meals will be a lot more interesting and tasty.

Aside from nutrition tables, use your common sense as the best guide to selecting the most beneficial foods for your diet. A simple rule is to avoid as much sugar and starch as possible and concentrate on vegetables, fruit, and animal and sea foods.

Chapter 11

Weight Control for Men: A Trimmer Figure in Thirty Days

In a scene from the 1960s film *Soldier in the Rain,* comedian Jackie Gleason stood in front of a full-length mirror trying unsuccessfully to rearrange his well-pressed army uniform around his bulging body. Finally giving it up as a bad job, he sighed wistfully, "It's not easy being a fat narcissist."

How right he is. Men generally look younger, more virile, and far more attractive when they're at their proper weight, yet more men today find themselves in Mr. Gleason's predicament. Aside from looks, overweight men aren't usually very healthy men. More die because of overweight than from smoking cigarettes. The problems associated with obesity include: overtiredness, shortness of breath, indigestion and constipation, headache, diabetes, inflammation of the gallbladder, cirrhosis of the liver, hernia, high blood pressure, varicose veins, kidney disease, greater operation risks, and a high mortality rate. The mortality rate for people more than 40 per cent overweight doubles that of the norm; just ask your insurance agent.

The diet recommended in this chapter has proved highly successful, not only for losing weight but for keeping it off permanently. The man shown in the photo section dropped sixty pounds in six months with his personal adaptation of it. You should see results within thirty days or less.

WHAT'S YOUR IDEAL WEIGHT?

Nutritionists don't know exactly what your "ideal" weight should be, but they have a good idea of the weight you should aim for. It's based upon the average weight of a great many well-proportioned, healthy men of your height. Of course there are exceptions for those at the extremes like professional Suma wrestlers and jockeys.

This table indicates the desirable weights for men of medium build, aged twenty-five years and over, in bare feet and naked.* Add seven pounds if you weigh yourself wearing shoes and indoor clothing.

HEIGHT		WEIGHT
ft.	*in.*	*pounds*
5	0	115–126
5	1	118–129
5	2	121–133
5	3	124–136
5	4	127–139
5	5	130–143
5	6	134–147
5	7	138–152

* Based upon figures from the Metropolitan Life Insurance Company.

5	8	142–156
5	9	146–160
5	10	150–165
5	11	154–170
6	0	158–175
6	1	162–180
6	2	167–185
6	3	172–190
6	4	177–195

If you're more than fifteen to twenty pounds above the maximum figure given for your height, you're almost certainly overweight regardless of your build. You may be on your way to overweight if you're only a few pounds outside the average.

Keep a twenty-year-old's figure. If you had a reasonably slim and trim figure in your twenties, a good rule of thumb is to keep to that weight for the rest of your life. I can't think of a legitimate reason for you to weigh much more than that, can you?

What causes your overweight?

Assuming a healthy body, the three major causes of overweight are overeating, eating the wrong types of food, and leading a less active life. Of course many of us claim other reasons which we'll discuss later under the heading of "The Myths of Weight Control."

You're overeating when your daily calorie intake exceeds the calories you burn up. This can differ from day to day depending upon your level of activity. Just twenty extra unburned calories a day (a little over one level teaspoon of sugar) can add about two pounds to your weight a year. Think of how much less you'd weigh today if you'd used saccharin in your coffee over the last five or ten years.

Some men burn more calories than others. Although not yet confirmed by research, it seems that with some lucky people, extra food stimulates their metabolism to burn up excess food. They can overeat without putting on weight. Men also differ in the efficiency with which their bodies use calories. The inefficient user burns more calories to do the same amount of work than his more efficient colleague. Therefore, he can afford to eat more than his friend without adding weight.

Pyschological factors play an important part in overeating. For some, food represents the security and love they had as children. Eating seems to comfort them under situations of stress and anxiety. Too many mothers stuff their children as proof of their love because they and their neighbors mistakenly regard plump children as healthy, happy children. The overeating habit sticks as the child grows older and fatter. Not too far removed, in some areas of the world obesity marks a wealthy man.

The wrong foods are high-calorie, low-nutritional foods containing lots of carbohydrates and fat, but little protein, vitamins, or minerals. These nutritionally inferior foods (such as sugar, bread, potatoes, wheat, rice, and other cereals) make up about 50 per cent of the diets in North America, Britain, and Western Europe which accounts, to some extent, for the high incidence of overweight in these countries.

Activity has surprisingly little effect on your weight. A sedentary life, with little physical activity, does lead to overweight unless you carefully restrict your intake of calories. Unfortunately, the reverse is not true. You can't rely upon exercise to keep your weight down.

The higher your level of activity, the more calories your body burns up—but also the hungrier you get. To satisfy this hunger, men often eat more calories than a particular exercise uses up. For example, one business lunch can nullify an eight-hour, nonstop game of squash. You'd have to swim seven hours or walk fifty miles in twenty hours to lose one pound of fat, and think of your appetite at the end of it all.

Exercise, in combination with a good weight-reducing diet, can help you lose weight. If you walk an extra half hour a day while on a diet, experts assure me that this added exercise will knock off an additional ten pounds a year on top of that lost due to your diet alone. Exercise also helps distribute weight more evenly and keeps up your muscle tone. Like wearing an invisible girdle, muscle can help keep your overweight midsection from sagging and becoming too obvious.

It may come as a surprise to you eggheads, but contrary to popular belief, increased amounts of mental activity need few extra calories. I'm afraid nuclear physicists can't use their work as an excuse for an extra helping of pudding.

AN EASY-TO-FOLLOW DIET FOR MEN THAT WORKS

This diet is based upon the very simple principle of cutting out the less nourishing, high-calorie, carbohydrate foods and concentrating on those rich in protein, vitamins, and minerals. It includes some fats, like butter, so that what you eat tastes good. In other words, you'll be eating less, but much better. Today many American and most British doctors advocate this type of low-carbohydrate diet or combine it with a low-fat diet as the best way to lose weight and keep it off.

I'm sure you'll agree that it meets all the criteria that make up the perfect diet for men.

1. **You lose weight.** Probably about half the calories in your present diet come from carbohydrates. Unlike protein and fats, the carbohydrate level in the average diet can be cut by seven-eighths without any threat to good health. Such a cut drastically reduces your daily calorie intake so that your body starts burning up its stored fat to meet its energy needs.

2. **It's nutritionally correct.** Your body will receive all the protein, fats, carbohydrates, vitamins, and minerals it needs for growth, maintenance, and health. By contrast, low-protein diets must be

adhered to strictly for health reasons and take weight off slowly. Calorie-counting diets can get you so involved in counting calories that you may neglect your nutritional needs.

3. **It's appetizing and easy to follow.** Crash diets and low-fat diets may enable you to drop some weight, but they're hard to follow, you're usually hungry all the time, and your meals aren't very appealing. When they're over, you drift back to bad eating habits and up goes your weight. Because it's easy and appetizing, this diet should change your tastes and eating habits so you become accustomed to eating sensibly and your weight loss will be permanent.

4. **It's socially practical.** Because of its flexibility, you can stick to this diet while having business lunches and dining socially without alienating the affections of every hostess in town by having to refuse her culinary masterpieces. In fact, most people won't even know you're watching your weight; they'll just consider you're one of the lucky men who are naturally slim.

How to make the low-carbohydrate diet work for you

Remember that to be really effective, a diet should be tailored to your individual needs, to the amount of weight *you* want to lose, the speed with which *you* want to lose it, and to *your* taste and eating habits. Therefore, approach this diet in four stages, going from one to the next to find the one best suited to you. If the first stage doesn't lose weight fast enough to satisfy you, go on to the more strict second stage or, with your doctor's permission, on to the third.

Stage 1: Simple elimination

First, make sure your current diet contains enough of the foods in each of the four groups discussed in the previous chapter for good nutrition. Now start eliminating carbohydrates from your diet in this order, with sugar and sweets the first to go.

1. Sugar and sweets
2. Pastry, puddings, and canned fruit

3. Bread, rolls, and pasta
4. Alcohol
5. Cereals, rice, and potatoes
6. Miscellaneous foods high in carbohydrates such as thick soups, nuts, dried fruit, condensed and evaporated milk (see the tables in Appendix 3).

Unlike the problems with other diets, there's little confusion about what you shouldn't eat, because you can easily recognize most high-carbohydrate foods, those sugar and starch foods. You don't have to worry much about the amounts of the noncarbohydrate foods you eat.

The more weight you want to lose, the more types of carbohydrate foods you should cut from your diet initially. (I cut out almost everything but some of the alcohol with great results.) Be patient. This diet usually takes about two to three weeks before having a significant effect on your weight; after that, the loss should be gradual and constant. If you've had no weight loss after a few weeks, you just haven't cut out enough carbohydrates, so eliminate several more types. It's a painless and relaxed way to lose and maintain your weight if you really follow through with it.

One of the advantages of this diet is that you'll automatically reduce your intake of fats (high in calories) without even trying, because by eliminating carbohydrates like bread and pastry, you've eliminated the vehicles responsible for transporting large amounts of fats, butter, and cream into your mouth. Thus you have some freedom to continue using butter on your vegetables, dressings on your salads, and cooking fats to make your meals more appetizing. Just use some discretion. You get another advantage from having some fat in your diet. Fat has a high satiety value, so you shouldn't be tormented by hunger pangs all day long.

The low-carbohydrate diet is practical and social because it contains most of the foods served you at dinners and you have some flexibility in eating carbohydrates. You probably won't offend your hostess very much by passing up a roll and her dessert, but if her heart looks like breaking, take the sweet and make up for it the next day by cutting extra carbohydrates. No great harm will have been done as long as you're honest with yourself.

STAGE 2: MAKE UP YOUR OWN DIET

If you want faster weight loss, you'll have to discipline yourself to more strict food control. This means restricting yourself to a fixed ration of carbohydrates each day.

Start with a basic diet of two reasonably sized portions (no need to measure or weigh) from each of the four food groups needed for good nutrition every day. Drink at least a glass (half pint) of milk a day.

Group 1	meat, fish, eggs
Group 2	milk, cheese
Group 3	fruit, vegetables
Group 4	butter, margarine

Now add only enough more food to make up your ration of carbohydrates. Of the foods in the four groups, only milk and a few vegetables and fruits contain enough carbohydrates to come into your calculations. (Appendix 3 contains the carbohydrate gram equivalents for various foods.) Start by rationing your intake to one hundred grams (your current diet probably contains about four hundred) on top of the basic diet. If you want to make a faster job of it, cut your ration to fifty grams, but not below. After a month or so, you'll be able to see the effect of the carbohydrate ration on your weight and can lower or raise the ration to suit the speed with which you want to lose weight.

Spend your ration on the foods that suit your taste and appetite. Fifty grams could be spent completely on diet luxuries like a pint of beer or a bloody mary (approximately twenty-five grams of carbohydrates), half an avocado (five grams), and a half cup of unsalted cashews (twenty grams). Or if you're less of a gourmet, have spaghetti with tomato and meat sauce (one cup at thirty-five grams) and a slice of rye bread (twelve grams). If you have a large appetite, increase the size of your meals by spending your fifty-gram ration on those foods with the least carbohydrate content.

Use the tables in Appendix 3 to get an idea of the carbohydrate content of various foods. The government puts out an excellent and detailed book on the composition of foods, and many commercial publications are available in bookstores.

Although we are dealing here with carbohydrate restriction, the basic object of this diet is to reduce calories. For this reason, at the same time you look up the carbohydrate values of foods, look at their calorie values and make a mental note of those common foods that are ridiculously high in calories. For example, a cup of cooked lima beans contains 140 calories, almost five times more than a cup of string beans, and so represents a rather poor choice. Once you've established these "poor choice" foods, you can forget calorie counting.

After the first two weeks on this strict diet, you should be losing at least two or three pounds a week.

STAGE 3: THE FORMAL LOW-CARBOHYDRATE DIET

If voluntary restrictions aren't helping you, then adopt the formal diet detailed in Appendix 2 with your doctor's approval. It contains only about 1,200 calories and is very effective. Surprisingly, this diet contains a variety of foods which makes it highly appetizing, so I don't think you'll find difficulty in sticking with it.

STAGE 4: MAINTAINING YOUR IDEAL WEIGHT

When you reach your best weight through dieting, be sensible. The purpose of this gradual weight-reducing diet is to retrain your eating habits so you won't miss the high-carbohydrate, high-calorie foods. You can ease up a bit on eating some of your favorite things, but don't go back on a sweet-and-starch binge. If you stick to essentially low-carbohydrate foods and weigh yourself weekly, you should be able to keep your new, more flattering figure.

Use sugar substitutes. If you've still got a sweet tooth, use saccharin to sweeten your coffee and food until you've conquered this addiction. Saccharin has no carbohydrates or calories. Be careful, however, about sugar "substitutes" in general, as some have almost as many calories as sugar itself.

Eat three meals a day, plus. The more often you eat, the more calories you burn up, because the same amount of exercise burns up more calories after eating than before. Don't eat extra food, but divide your daily intake between the three basic meals and snacks.

Give in to the urge to eat between meals, but nibble raw vegetables or a bit of cheese. Cheese has only a trace of carbohydrate and contains fat which reduces hunger pangs. But don't go overboard.

Breakfast gives you morning energy and also lowers your appetite for lunch. Don't take dinner so late that you haven't time to burn calories with some activity before going to bed. It would be best to have your main meal at midday. (Unfortunately, the more times you eat, the worse for your teeth. So eat *and* brush.)

Have dry martinis instead. If you're weight watching, go easy on alcohol. You have enough carbohydrates in your ration to afford a drink or two if you scrimp the rest of the day, but beware of the mixers. Some, like tonic, have a lot of calories, so have a martini and drink your whiskey neat, with water or club soda.

Dry wine contains fewer carbohydrates and calories than sweet wine and fewer than hard liquor. Many people now drink only dry wine at cocktail parties. Not only does it help their waists, but they drive home more safely.

Combine exercise and diet. For you who lead a very sedentary life, an increase in daily activity will help your body regulate its appetite and proper food intake. Climb a few extra flights of stairs, try to walk an extra half hour a day, and walk to the next bus stop, not the closest one.

How to weigh yourself. You'll be encouraged only if you get on the scales and see your lost weight has stayed lost, so weigh yourself sensibly:

- Always use the same scales.
- Always weigh yourself naked or with the same type of clothing.
- Weigh at the same time of day.
- Weigh yourself only once a week, as your weight can vary from day to day for different reasons.

ADD WEIGHT IF NECESSARY

This chapter has dealt with losing weight; some of you, like the scrawny man on the beach in the muscle-building ads, may feel the need to put more flesh on your bones and fill out your build.

To do this, concentrate on eating body-building foods, not fat-making ones. Eat lots of protein and minerals in addition to your normal, varied diet. Draw heavily from the four basic food groups recommended for proper nutrition.

Try dietary (not appetite-reducing) biscuits, cookies, or drinks between regular meals. As many of these biscuits or liquids were designed to supply most of your body's daily nutrient needs, you'll be greatly increasing your intake of body-building material.

Weight-adding branded products may be of help to you, so get your doctor's advice concerning their advantages and how best to combine them with your regular diet. Also consult him concerning the use of male hormone (anabolic steroids) injections which, in conjunction with diet, can add many pounds of muscle bulk in a relatively short time. Muscle builders often use them, but they have disadvantages.

THE MYTHS OF WEIGHT CONTROL

I was recently rebuked by a very overweight Parisian who claimed that the phrase "excuses for obesity" implied that overweight was bad, something that needed to be excused, and that I would build guilt complexes in the readers of this book. He went on to justify his weight by heredity, glands, and water retention while pouring himself another drink.

At the risk of building guilt complexes, let's dispose of some of the excuses—not to mention manufacturers' claims—confusing weight control. If you decide you need to lose weight, don't spend a lot of money, time, and effort on things that won't do the job for you. Remember, there's no easy way; you can't slim without dieting.

Sweating off weight

A pint of water weighs one and a quarter pounds. It's quite true that getting rid of some water by sweltering in Turkish baths or exercising in plastic suits will reduce your weight—temporarily. You're not getting rid of fat, just water.

Up to three fourths of your body consists of water. When dehydrated, it will try to regain its natural water balance by replacing the water you've sweated off from your normal intake of liquids and food. If you want to go thirsty for days, you'll drop weight, but like a camel, you have to drink sometime.

Salt-free diets cut weight, but . . .

In health, the salt within your body helps regulate the amount of water your body retains and its distribution. Restricting salt in your diet can lower your body's water content, but can be unhealthy unless closely supervised by a doctor.

As it's rare for water retention to be a major cause of obesity, why disturb a healthy body's important water and salt balance? It's about as logical as lopping off an arm to reduce your over-all weight.

Can special garments redistribute weight and slim you?

Ads for a variety of knickers, armlets, waist belts, etc., imply they melt away fat and redistribute it throughout your body to reapportion it and make you look slimmer. Remember, fat disappears when it's burned up, not melted.

In 1958 *Which?*, the Consumer Association's publication in Britain, stated in their opinion these types of garments were not effective and challenged their manufacturers to prove their claims scientifically. Ten years later that challenge had not yet been accepted.

Does massage reduce weight?

Your masseur may lose some of *his* weight, but *your* fat reserves won't dissolve or vanish by being bashed about; your body must burn them up. It has been proved that a pressure of between fifty and seventy-five pounds per square inch must be exerted to break up fat cells. With such pressure, the injury to your body tissue would be extreme.

How about machine-induced exercise?

Like massage, being twitched by electric shocks, vibrated by belts, and undertaking similar forms of passive exercise won't dissolve fat. Unfortunately, time spent on these pursuits won't even help your muscles much.

If you want to improve the shape of your body by strengthening its surrounding girdle of muscles, you'll have to engage in active physical exercise.

"But I have big bones"

You can't excuse overweight by attributing it solely to big bones. Bones comprise about one sixth of the total weight of a well-proportioned trim man. If 160 pounds represents the average weight for your height and build, your bones should weigh about 27 pounds. Assuming your weight tops 180 pounds, it's impossible for all 20 pounds of extra weight to be the fault of your bones. They can't possibly weigh that much.

Can glands be blamed?

Only in part can glands be blamed. Glands, like your thyroid, pituitary, and suprarenal glands, are concerned with your metabolism. Many people with too much thyroid hormone remain thin and can be said to metabolize fast, while others with insufficient thyroid seem to metabolize too slowly and tend toward fat.

But much of the weight problem still goes back to overeating. Slow metabolizers don't burn food quickly and therefore don't need as much. If they eat just what their bodies require, they don't put on weight. As proof, more than half of those short of thyroid aren't overweight.

Only rarely do glands deserve the sole blame for obesity, so if people stop using them as a convenient excuse and try to adjust their food intake to their rate of metabolism, they should lose weight.

Heredity as a scapegoat

Your metabolism, the efficiency with which you use calories, and other inherited factors do play a part in overweight. But just because your family is fat, if you watch your diet, you don't necessarily have to be fat as well.

Identical twins raised separately both tend to overweight. If brought up together, that tendency becomes greater. This leads to the importance of environment. We aren't born with our eating habits, but learn most of them. We usually eat the sorts and amounts of foods our parents eat, and pass these habits on to our children. Fat-making eating habits can make generations of fat relatives unless those habits undergo a change. One of the grossest men I've ever known used to joke about the "amusing" little poem with which his parents blessed their food at mealtimes:

God bless us all, if we are able,
To lift our bellies 'bove the table.

CHAPTER 12

Sex: Virility Plus Fertility Equals Conception

What's sex all about? Most men claim to know a lot more about it than they really do, and so some suffer under misconceptions that bring them frustration and grief. Having good sex and building the right-sized family depends on knowing how and when to have intercourse. It also depends on keeping up your virility and fertility as long as possible.

Your role in conception is to produce and deliver sperm to the right place at the right time. You should be sufficiently fertile to manufacture the proper amounts of healthy spermatozoa and sufficiently virile to hold an erection long enough to penetrate your wife and ejaculate the sperm at the entrance to her uterus. This should be done during her most fertile period, and the act itself should give you both a lot of pleasure.

THE STEPS TO CONCEPTION

Keeping up your erection

You get an erection because erotic stimulation causes blood to flow into the spongy tissue in your penis to swell and harden it. If you have difficulty, you might try applying an irritant preparation to your glans which gives added stimulation to help you hold an erection. From experience, I'm sure you know that too much alcohol, tranquilizing drugs, or similar relaxants can make it hard to sustain an erection, so watch them.

The "cock ring" is another aid to keeping an erection. This adjustable metal or plastic ring tightly encircles the base of your penis and testicles to inhibit the flow of blood back out of your penis. Be careful where you wear it, though. Not long ago a prominent executive on his way to Washington was stopped by the buzzing of a New York airport's electronic weapon detector. As an interested crowd looked on, security guards asked him to empty his pockets of all change and keys: the unfortunate man wasn't carrying any. A few knowing smiles flickered across the faces of the more sophisticated onlookers, and the sympathetic guard waved our crimson-faced friend through. He'd worn his metal cock ring in anticipation of going directly from the plane to his mistress's flat. Chalk one up to experience.

Producing healthy sperm

Spermatozoa start life in the **seminiferous tubules** of your **testicles.** They continue to mature and develop "motility" (their capacity for spontaneous movement) as they pass through the **epididymis** and move on up your **vas deferens.** Finally they reach the **ampullar section** of your vas where they're stored for future use.

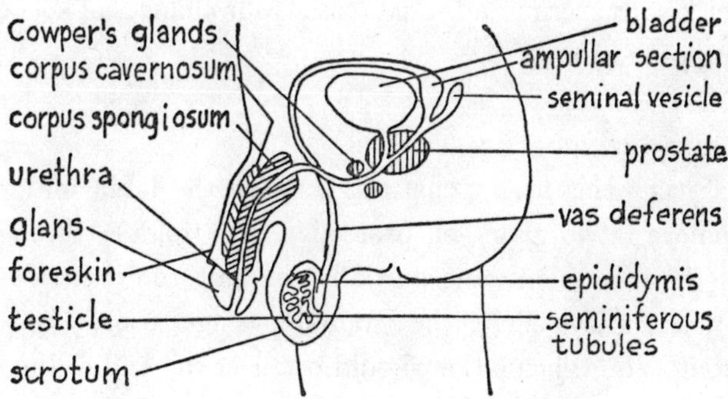

It takes about ten weeks for your testes to make mature sperm and an additional three weeks for it to move up to the ampullar section—a total of about three months. You'll see later how this affects your fertility. By the time it reaches freedom, each microscopic spermatozoon has traveled through some thirty-four feet of tubes and pipes.

What is semen?

Semen is a mixture of your sperm and liquids that nourish, protect, and act as a vehicle for it. When you ejaculate, the **Cowper's glands** starts off by releasing a small bit of mucus; next your **prostate gland** secretes a thin, opalescent fluid containing calcium and citrate. Then comes the sperm, and finally your **seminal vesicles** loose the largest part of the semen, an alkaline fluid containing the fructose the spermatozoa need for spontaneous movement (their motility).

A normal ejaculation contains about a teaspoon of semen. Depending upon the frequency of ejaculation, it has between 300 and 400 million spermatozoa in it. If you have sex three times a day for two days, your semen will have relatively little sperm left on the third day. Sexual abstinence for several days can result in semen being thick with sperm, and so increases your chances of successfully fertilizing your wife.

The path to conception

Your erect penis must penetrate between the **labia majora** and **labia minora** (two pairs of protective skin folds), through the **hymen** (the thin membrane partially covering the entrance of the vagina), and move along the **vaginal passage,** usually some four inches long. Your ejaculation should occur at the end of the vagina at the **cervix,** the constricted neck of the **uterus** (womb).

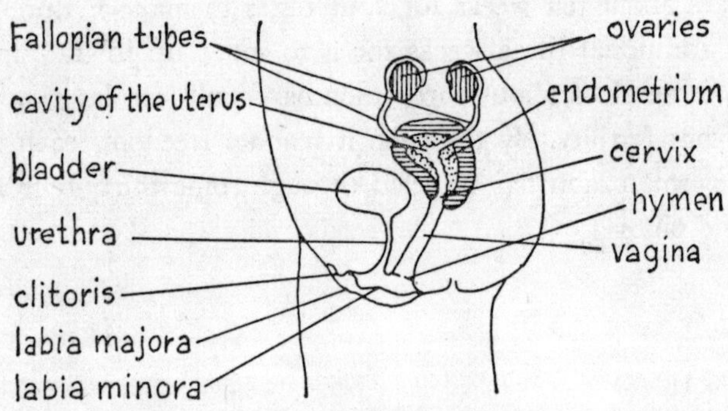

Many of your freed sperm swim into the uterus (some within ninety seconds) and move along its walls. A few find their way up the **fallopian tubes** where hopefully one meets and fertilizes an **ovum** (egg) moving down from the **ovary.** Sperm can remain alive for about two days inside a woman's body.

What's the best time for conception?

The best time for conception is at ovulation, about fourteen days before the start of the woman's next menstrual period. The average menstrual cycle runs some twenty-eight days, although it can vary from twenty to forty days. Few women menstruate with complete regularity. During the first half of her cycle, the ovaries release increasing amounts of estrogen hormones into the bloodstream which encourages the lining of the uterus (the **endometrium**) to thicken in readiness to receive a fertile ovum.

At puberty your wife's ovaries hold many thousands of follicles. About fourteen days before the end of each cycle, one follicle reaches maturity, bursts, and ejects an ovum through the covering layer of the ovary so it will fall into a fallopian tube. During her productive years, the average woman will shed only about four hundred ova, one at a time, through this process called ovulation. After releasing the ovum, the follicle produces progesterone hormones which combine with the estrogen to continue the thickening of the endometrium.

Her ovum moves slowly down its fallopian tube (about four inches long) for two days. If during that time it meets one of your spermatozoa, fertilization can take place. Your spermatozoon contains an enzyme which breaks down part of the ovum's outer cover so it can penetrate it and start the complex exchange of genetic material with her ovum.

When fertilized, the ovum "telegraphs" this fact back to the ovary which starts producing increased quantities of estrogen and progesterone to further build the uterus lining. After leaving the fallopian tube, the ovum takes a day or two to imbed itself in the prepared lining of the uterus where it continues to develop into a fetus. Menstruation ceases.

If her ovum hasn't been fertilized while in the tube, a woman's level of hormone production drops toward the end of the cycle causing her to menstruate, to shed the endometrium along with mucus and blood for three to eight days. Her uterus, thus cleaned, becomes ready for a new cycle to begin.

CHAPTER 13

Virility: How to Keep It Up

Virility refers to your mental character: vigorous, strong, initiative, and confidently assertive. It refers in exactly the same way to your attitude toward sex and your physical capacity to engage in it. In other words, can you get it up and keep it up—as often as you'd like. Unfortunately, a man usually reaches the peak of his virility between the ages of fifteen and twenty, whereas a woman is fully developed sexually and most likely to be interested in sex at about thirty-five. This may account for so much tea and sympathy between older women and younger men. Sexually, a man begins to decline around the age of thirty-five; it becomes noticeable at forty-five and certain at fifty-five.

With age, your penis becomes less stiff and its angle of erection lowers. The duration of your erection shortens, and it takes longer for you to ejaculate. Interest in sex also declines. But don't despair—there are some simple and pleasant ways to pep up lagging virility.

INCREASE YOUR VIRILITY

Increase your sex activity

The old phrase "The more you get, the more you want" is quite true scientifically. Your glands produce hormones during intercourse which stimulate your appetite for the next session. The more sex you have, the more you can have.

If you're sexually active, you'll probably have a great desire for more after three days of abstinence. A man with a low level of activity won't miss sex for a much longer time. As a wonderful old doctor in Texas said when asked if too much sex could be harmful, "Son, it ain't never gonna wear out, but it sure as hell will rust out."

Be more imaginative

Have you ever had the feeling of "Oh, God . . . the same bed, same woman, same position; wonder what's on TV"? Boredom dulls virility just as it does your other senses. Stimulate your sexual desire with someone or something new: the excitement of the chase, the doubts of "will she or won't she," the triumph of a seduction well executed, new sex techniques or positions, props—they all help. Try the lot.

Many unhappy couples with inhibited attitudes toward sex have been helped by discussions and/or treatment aimed at getting them to regard sex more for its complete animal enjoyment than as something that's not very nice which you do to have babies and relieve tension. This new attitude leads to sexual inventiveness, new stimulations, increased excitement, and mutual virility. One swinging couple panic a bit whenever they pass through customs on vacation. They're embarrassed that one particular suitcase with its mysterious contents (they won't tell anyone if it's chains, whips, drag, or what) might fall under prudish scrutiny of a local customs inspector.

Keep fit

Good physical condition has a positive effect upon your virility. Conversely, being overtired or working to exhaustion may sometimes lead to temporary impotence. After healthy activity, sportsmen often have increased sex drives and capacities. This could account for the wild enthusiasm of the "après ski." Get thee to the slopes.

Try an aphrodisiac

Do aphrodisiacs really exist? Yes, though not in quite the way you may think. Here's a list I was given by a doctor in a major research complex working with hormones and sex drives:

- Anything you think an aphrodisiac becomes an aphrodisiac. Whether it's olives, oysters, or ostrich eggs, if you believe in its mystic powers, your mind will overcome your matter and up you'll go.
- Alcohol, marijuana, and hashish act as aphrodisiacs because they lower your inhibitions toward jumping into bed with anyone, or in some cases, anything. They may lead to more aggressive, imaginative, and thus more virile sex play. Obviously, too much of the three can leave you with the desire, but not the ability. Even worse you might fall asleep.
- Stay away from Spanish fly (cantharides). It's technically not an aphrodisiac, but a dangerous drug which irritates your bladder and kidneys. The drug causes an itchy sensation in the genital tract and sometimes congests the erectile tissues, but these sensations aren't accompanied by an improvement in your sexual desires or performance.
- Although your wife may not approve, variety is the best aphrodisiac of all. Men's blood pressure usually rises more dur-

ing extramarital intercourse than during sex with their wives. If you can't play the field, find some ways of jazzing things up at home.

See a psychiatrist

Psychological causes represent a man's most common causes of impotency. Anxiety, exaggerated timidity, lack of confidence, and a variety of other complexes can often be eased or so treated that potency is restored. If you even suspect this problem, discuss it with your doctor: you probably won't be the first one to consult him on this subject.

Hormone transplants and injections

Men over sixty may have their libido greatly increased by implants or injections of the testosterone hormone. Your body's manufacture of these hormones decreases with age and thus, so does your virility. Hormone implants and injections may have kept many an aging and famous personality chasing the girls.

Further investigations into artificial hormones may come up with effective and easier ways of achieving "instant virility." American scientists are now testing an artificial hormone that supposedly turns male houseflies into sex maniacs, sexually assaulting everything that moves. It's hoped that they'll burn themselves out and lose all interest in sex, thus cutting down the fly population. What next?

WHAT ATTRACTS WOMEN TO YOU?

All too many men blow their seductions because they don't really know what turns a woman on. Because of the current confusion surrounding unisex and maleness, they fall back on the traditional stereotypes of masculinity to impress their chums and attract women. Unfortunately, they understand better what impresses their chums than what appeals to women.

Tradition says that to be a masculine man you've got to drive your car faster, drink more, occasionally smash up the place, succeed in business, thrive on danger, and take risks. How many men do you know that still behave this way and go out of their way to tell you about it? Psychologists might say they're overcompensating for some real or imagined hang-up. With the exception of business success, apparently few women find anything attractive or appealing about the other traits.

What do women find appealing in men? Hold your hats. Tarzan and Jane wouldn't make it at all today. Two small polls conducted by the *Village Voice** in New York City made a comparison between the parts of the clothed male anatomy that one hundred men thought most turned women on, and those male parts that one hundred women actually admitted did turn them on. The results of the two polls were in almost complete disagreement:

	What women said most appealed to them	*What men thought appealed to women*
Buttocks (usually described by women as small and sexy)	39%	4%
Slimness	15%	7%
Flat stomach	13%	9%
Eyes	11%	4%
Long legs	6%	3%
Hair texture (not length)	5%	4%
Tallness	5%	13%
Neck	3%	2%

* Research conducted by Howard Smith and Tracy Young.

Penis (as suggested by tight trousers)	2%	15%
Muscular chest and shoulders	1%	21%
Muscular arms	0%	18%

In addition, these women listed a man's voice, manners, mode of dress, and possibly his little-boy-lost charm as important "turn-ons." Discussion with others indicated the appeal of a man's intelligence, sensitivity, warmth, and similar qualities as well as some of the traditional, but less boisterous, traits of confidence, courage, and honor. This gives you quite a lot of scope in luring your dream girl to bed. Good luck.

CHAPTER 14

Fertility: How to Increase Yours

The man bears responsibility for a couple's infertility in about half of the cases investigated. Fortunately, infertility isn't necessarily permanent. There are ways you can increase it.

Your fertility should remain more or less constant up to the age of forty. It can last, although in ever diminishing levels, until you're sixty, seventy, or older. Living sperm has been found in the semen of ninety-year-olds.

Your production of healthy sperm depends upon a delicate and stable balance between your glands and testicles, and their environment. Various factors can increase or decrease this production and your fertility. Here they are.

IMPROVING FERTILITY

KEEP YOUR TESTICLES COOL

When Cole Porter sang "It's too damn hot," he knew what he was singing about. Heat can be a major cause of infertility. Your

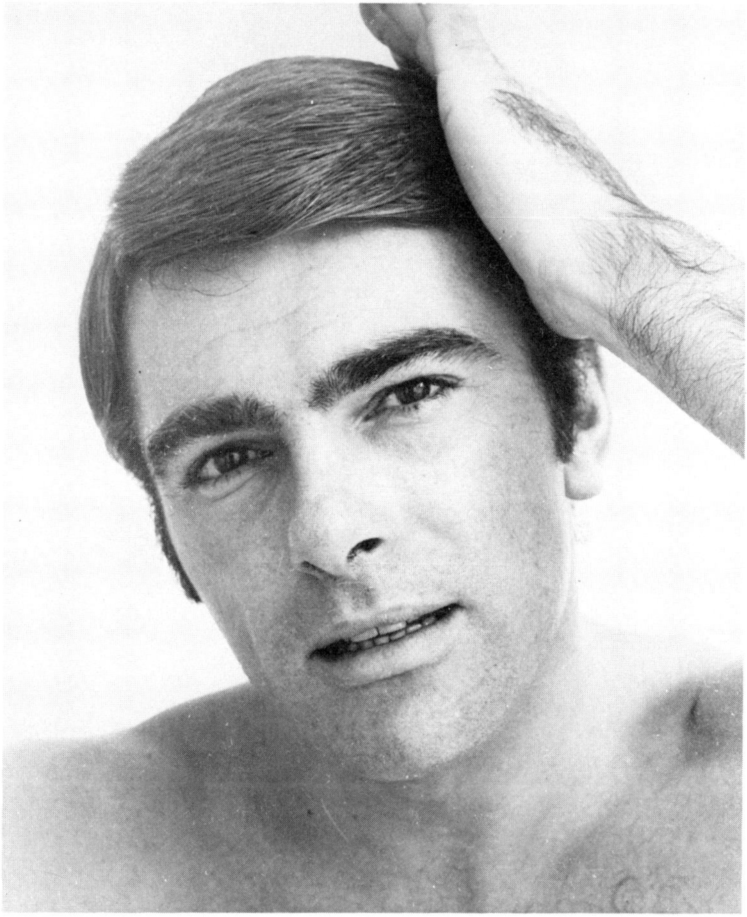

Hard-to-handle hair can easily be controlled and waved with a water set, net, and dryer.

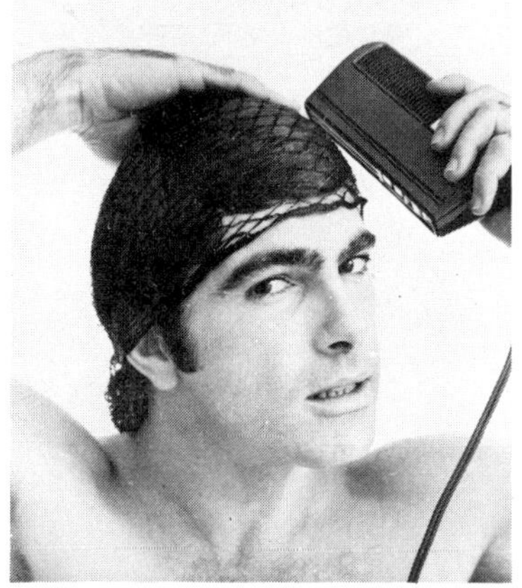

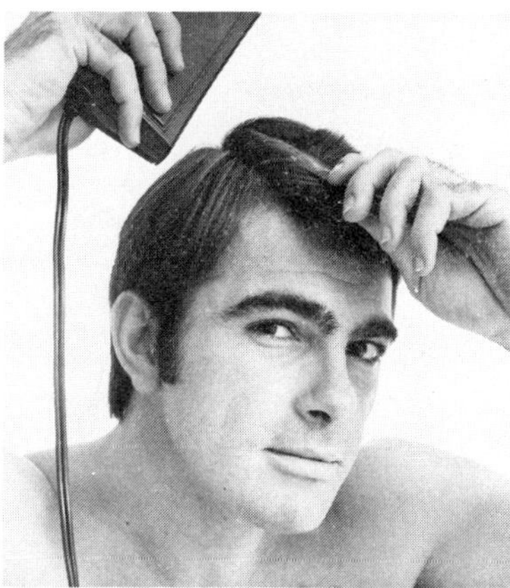

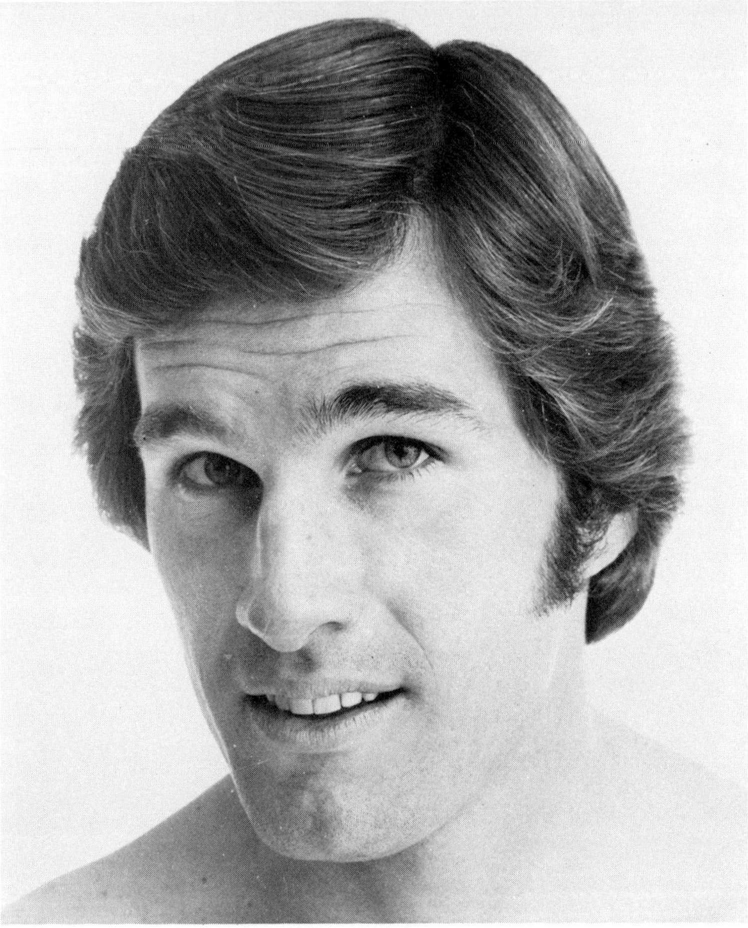

Style more manageable hair with a dryer and keep it in place with a light spray.

Younger man applying hair spray.

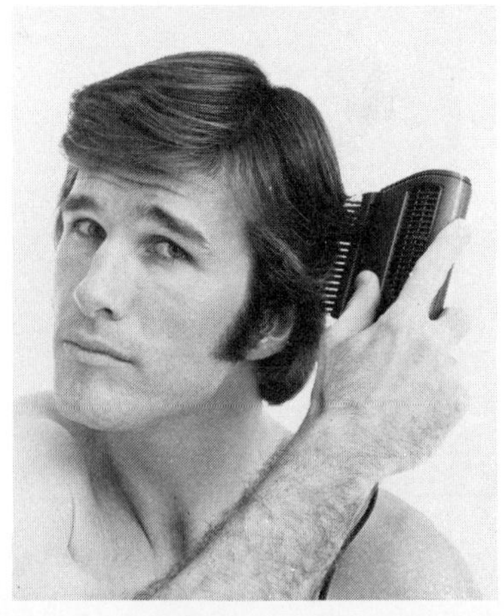

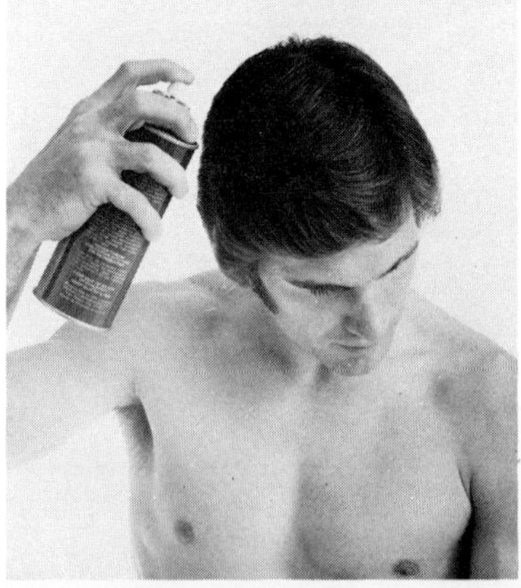

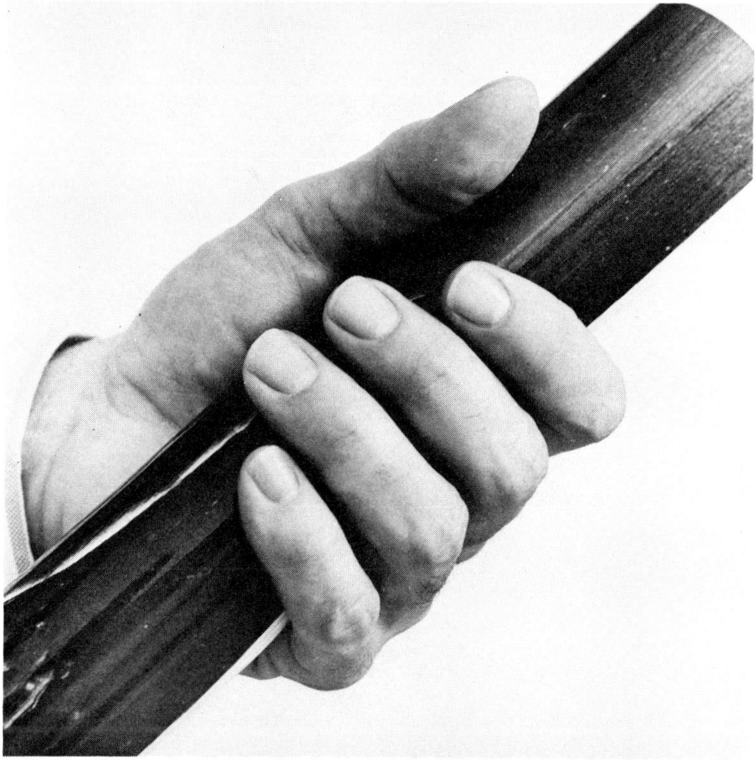

Restore smooth cuticles by lifting them with a hoofstick; don't push them back. Trim away hangnails with clippers.

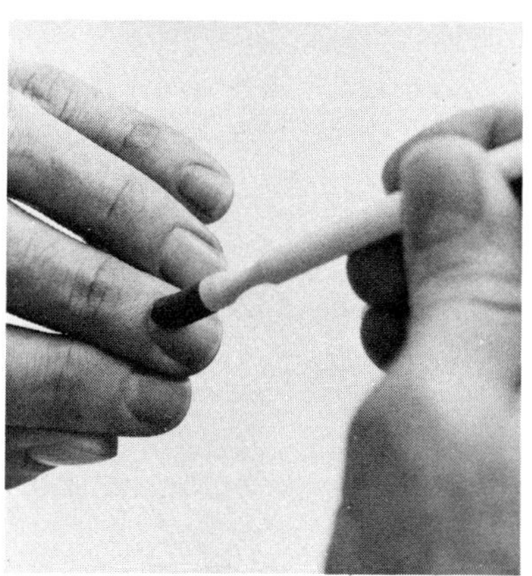

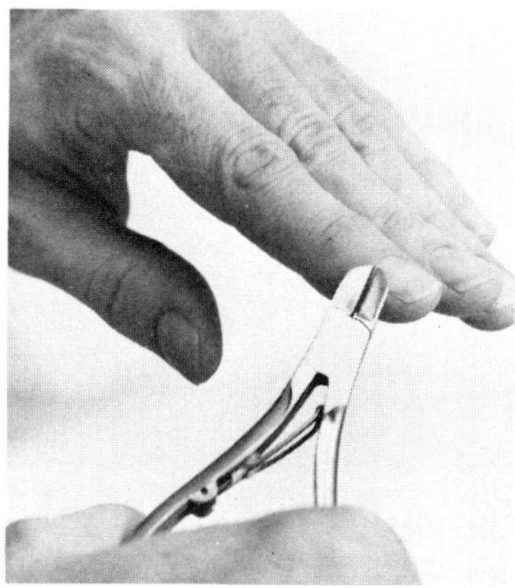

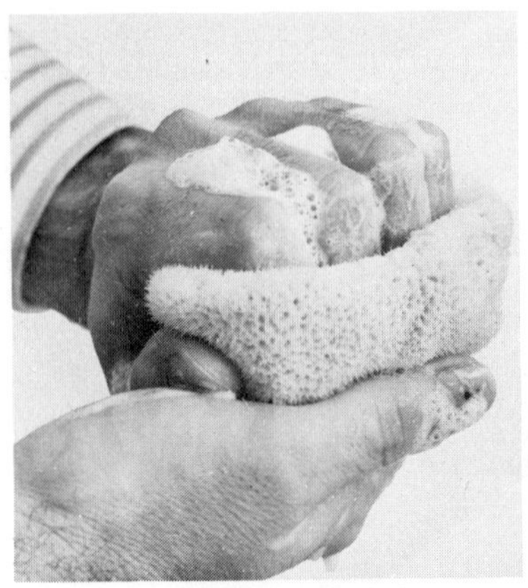
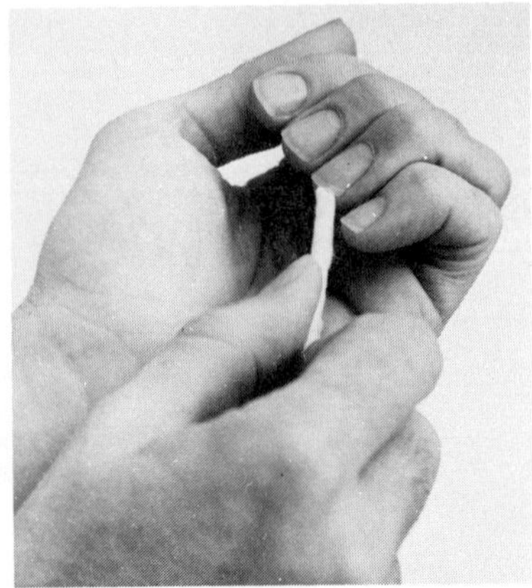

Use a cup sponge and an orange stick wrapped in cotton to remove dirt from under the nails.

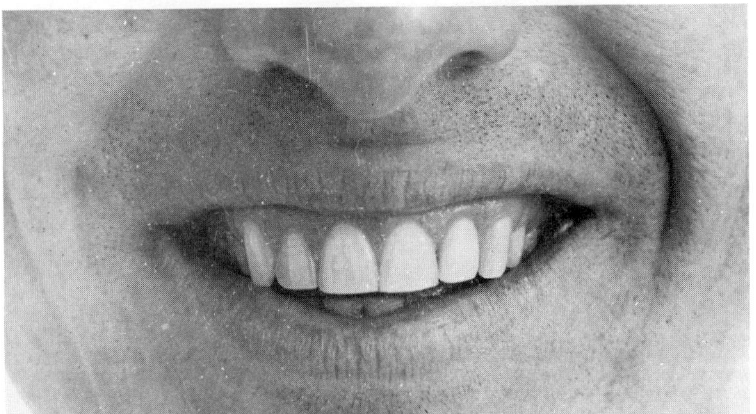

Nine weeks ago the three center teeth were overcrowded and crooked. A removable brace will be worn at night until the teeth become firmly anchored in their realigned position.

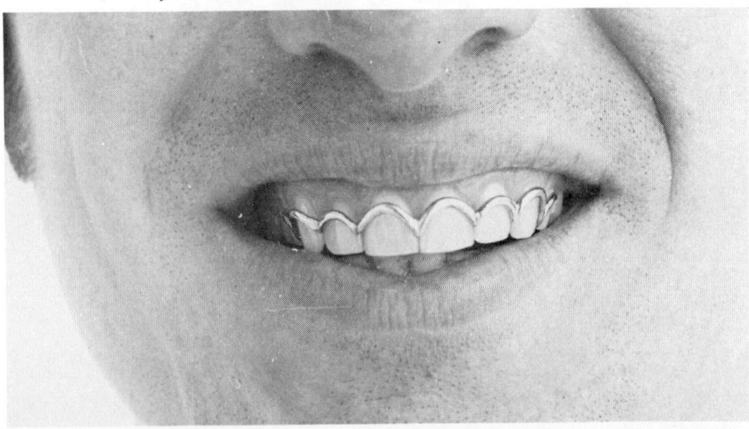

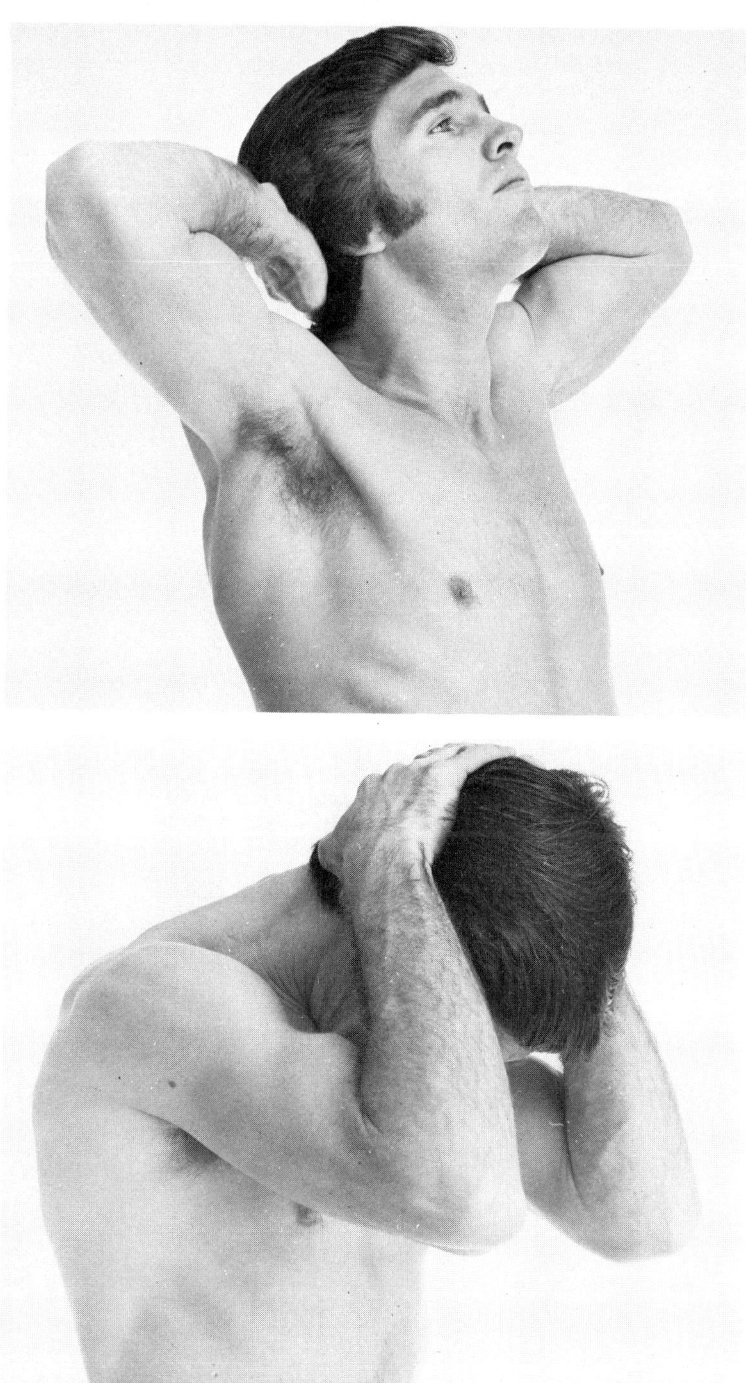

This isometric exercise strengthens the neck and shoulder muscles for better posture and relief of upper back and neck aches.

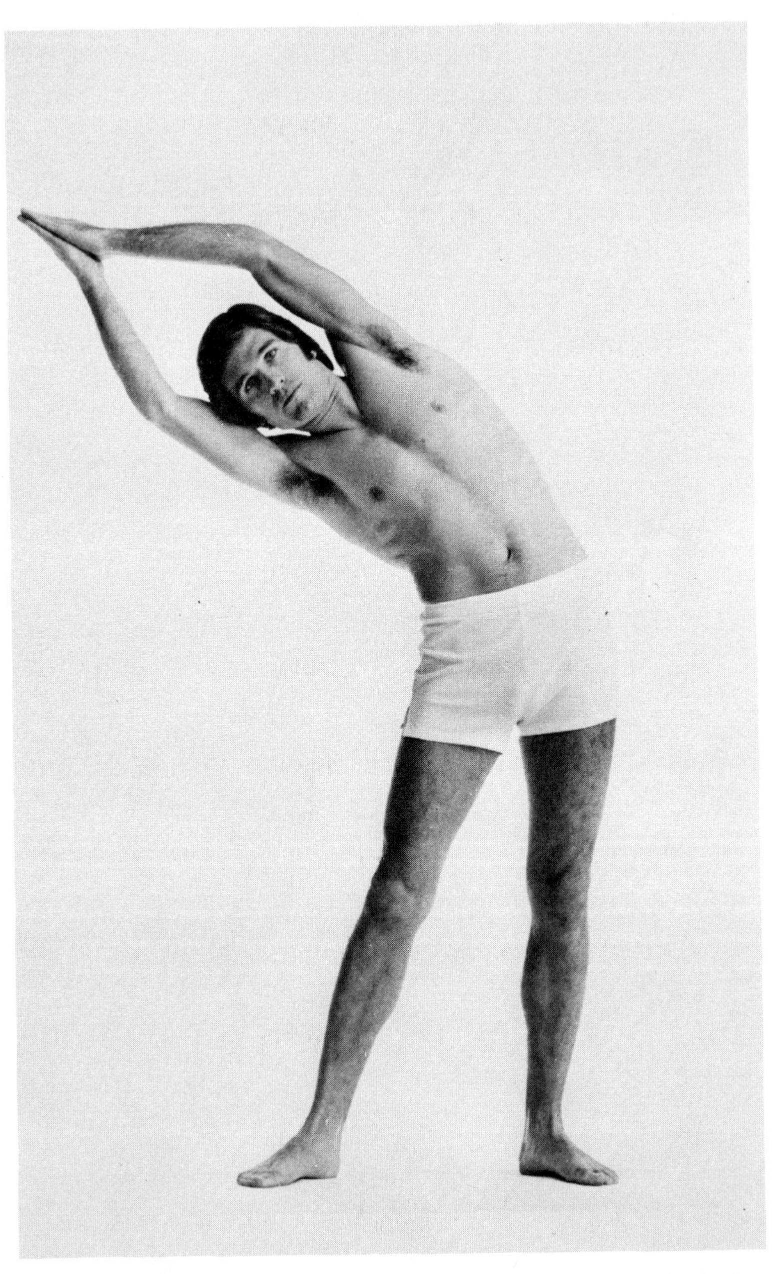

This man lost sixty pounds in six months on a low carbohydrate diet. The exercise strengthens the lower back muscles and keeps the waist trim.

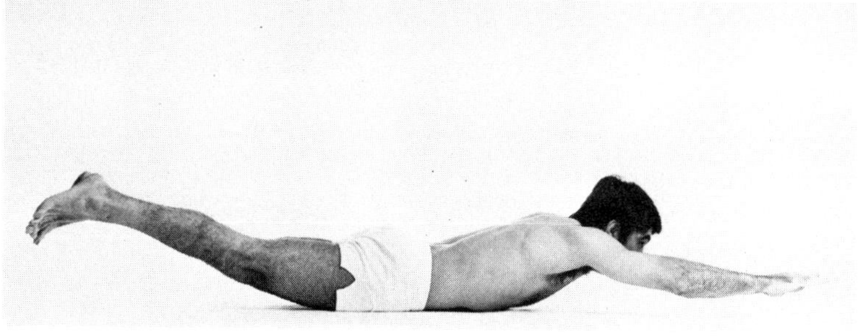

The Spine Extension exercise (above) and the "U" exercise (below) strengthen the girdle muscles supporting the spine in its proper position.

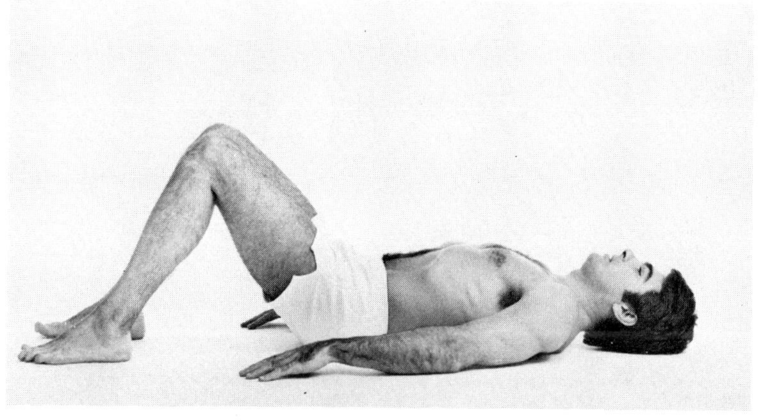

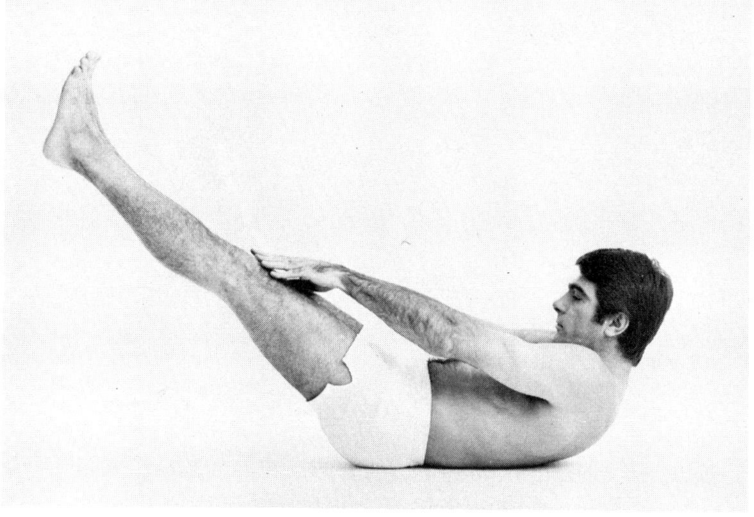

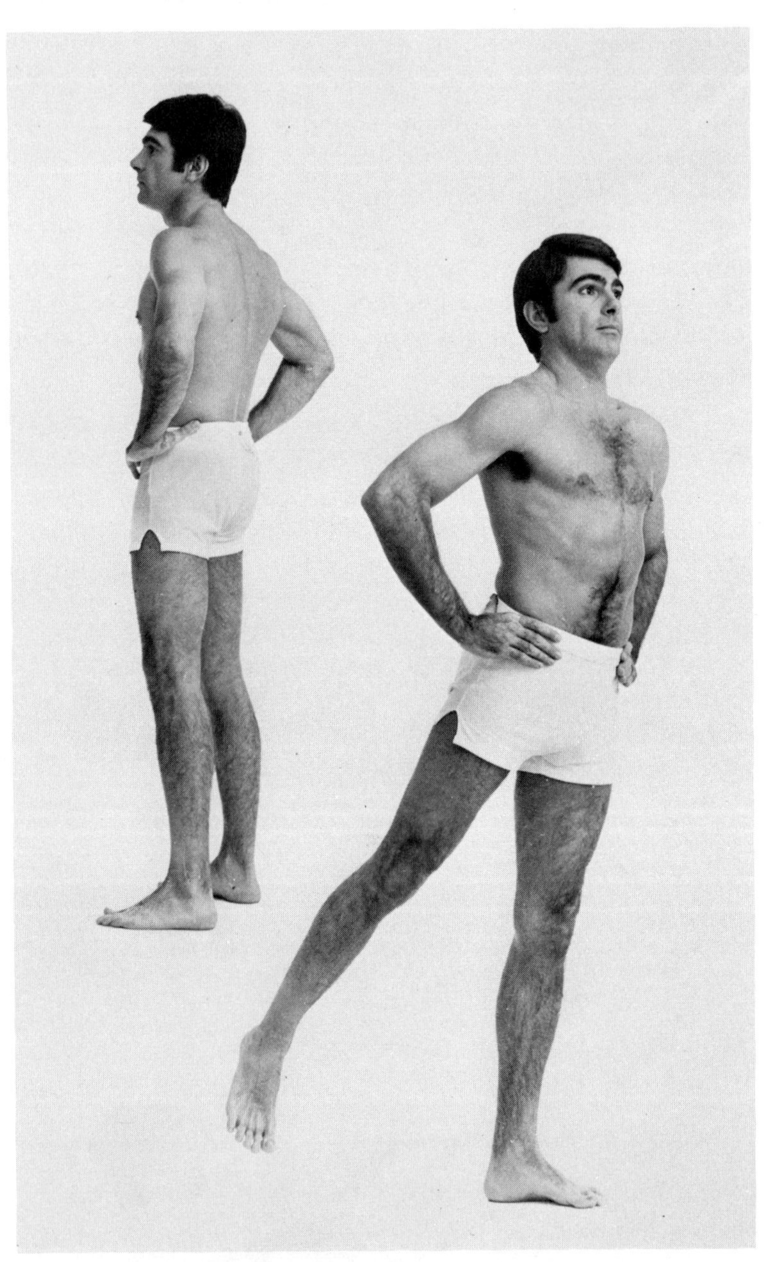

This leg-stretching exercise also firms up the buttocks. Proper posture eliminates much of the strain on the lower spine.

testicles function effectively at almost 4 degrees Fahrenheit below that of your intra-abdominal temperature. That's why they hang outside your body in the scrotum where they're kept cool. If you expose them to temperatures equal to or higher than your body's for any significant length of time, you'll lower or stop sperm production. This process can generally be reversed by restoring their temperature to its proper level, and within three months your sperm count should be back to normal. (An exception to this occurs in cryptochism, where one or both testes fail to fall naturally through the body's muscle layer into the cooler scrotum. If not in the scrotum by the age six, fertility can be irreversibly affected. If not there by puberty, a testicle will never be capable of sperm production. In these cases the testicles can be pulled down physically by a surgeon.)

There are many sources of heat that adversely affect your fertility. Most of these can be avoided or corrected.

Wear loose underpants. The ancient Chinese fasten a small, impermeable box over their testicles to increase the temperature as a means of contraception. Tight-fitting undergarments, jockstraps (particularly with protective plastic or metal cups), and form-clinging trousers can have the same marginal effect by pressing your testes close against your warm abdomen and inhibiting scrotal ventilation.

If you've been wearing tight, Y-front underwear for ten years or so, a switch to more ventilated ones like boxer shorts should get you back into normal sperm production within several weeks. If you haven't been wearing them very long, it may only take a few days to restore normal production.

Watch your weight. Obesity may limit fertility in cases where the fat of the thighs and abdomen encroaches on the testes to inhibit good ventilation.

Avoid high fevers. This may be like saying, "Stop getting colds." Illnesses accompanied by extremely high fever can cause temporary decline in fertility. Studies of volunteers subjected to fever treatment showed lower sperm level counts from twenty-five to fifty-five days after treatment. Full recovery occurred within three months in all cases. If you do get one of these illnesses, take very good care of yourself to reduce the fever as quickly as possible.

Take hot baths, if you want. Some people attribute the fall of Rome to all the hot baths they took, but you can forget this wacky explanation of history. As sperm production continues twenty-four hours a day, the temporary raising of testicle temperature for a few minutes in a hot bath or shower would have only a very brief effect on production. To kill mature sperm stored in your vas, the water would have to be so hot that you'd die as well.

Hygiene hasn't any effect on virility unless an unclean or smelly body turns off your bed partner, which it probably will. So regardless of the old wives' tales against washing before sex—bathe and ball.

Eat well

A balanced diet should supply all the requirements you need to maintain good fertility without worry. Only extreme nutritional deficiencies can temporarily affect it, and you'll probably never have this problem.

We've all heard a lot, if not too much, about the supposed effects of vitamin E on a man's sex life. It's true that a study on rats showed that an absence of this vitamin caused irreversible damage to their fertility. To date, however, I've not been able to find any undisputed proof that the controversial vitamin E has any significant effect on improving the fertility or virility of men.

Keep healthy

Mumps is the most destructive infection that can hit your testicles after puberty. It may inflame them and, when severe, damage their sperm-producing cells. In most cases only one testicle is involved, and if enlarged during the illness, you have a fifty-fifty chance of some degree of reduction in your fertility. If both suffer, sterility can result. Accute viral illnesses like **hepatitis** and **mononucleosis** may cause temporary, but often significant, reduction in fertility.

An extreme **emotional shock** can sometimes cause temporary reduction in your sperm production. **Diabetic men** have an unusually high rate of impotence. **Allergic reactions** to some drugs may cause temporary infertility and so can some antidepressants and drugs like heroin and cocaine, if only because they greatly reduce sexual desire. Studies are under way to discover drugs or agents that suppress male fertility for possible use in a contraceptive pill.

Stay away from x-ray equipment

Radiation can have harmful effects on your testicles and you should shield them from exposure, particularly if you're a doctor, dentist, or technician using radiation equipment. At one time unshielded shoe salesmen, using fluoroscopes to demonstrate well-fitted shoes, developed fertility problems.

Testosterone treatments may help

Although testosterone hormones have an inhibiting effect on sperm manufacture, they can sometimes be used to increase fertility temporarily. When given in a series of injections for several weeks to subfertile men, the hormone initially reduces production. When the treatments stop, a rebound reaction may occur giving a temporary rise in sperm production which enables successful conception.

Correct physical and psychological disorders

Inherited defects in the sperm-producing machinery can cause varying degrees of infertility. The different tubes and ducts along which the spermatozoa must travel may become blocked or separated by infection or injury. Surgery often repairs these problems.

Operate to correct varicose veins surrounding your spermatic cord and testicles. They can reduce fertility by raising the temperature of the testes with the increased amount of warm blood flowing past and/or by carrying potentially inhibiting toxins to your testicles. The problem is usually corrected by surgery.

A painfully tight foreskin, a deformed urethra opening, or an unusual curve to the penis may make it difficult or impossible for a man to carry on intercourse properly. These disorders can usually be cured surgically.

Premature ejaculation as well as failure to ejaculate are usually conditions of psychogenic origin and can often be cured through psychotherapy.

DO YOU HAVE A FERTILITY PROBLEM? OR YOUR WIFE?

There's usually no problem in producing children if both you and your wife are normally fertile or one of you is subfertile while the other is highly fertile. If you two are under thirty but haven't been able to produce a pregnancy after a year of regular intercourse without contraception, seek medical advice. So, too, should older couples if they've not been successful after six months of effort or if they're having trouble getting a second child ("second infertility"). Of course there's no need to wait for help if you're anxious.

Testing fertility

To determine the reason for infertility and which of you is responsible, your doctor or gynecologist will most certainly investigate the following areas:

1. The age and general health of you both and your medical histories to find any operations, illness, VD or other infection which may have affected fertility.
2. Your occupation from the standpoint of tension and stress and to determine if your job's location, demands, or

working hours interfere with regular intercourse by making it difficult or inconvenient.

3. Your frequency of intercourse, any difficulties experienced, and the positions you and your wife use.

4. The knowledge you both have concerning her period of highest fertility, menstrual cycles, and so forth. Often infertility can be laid to basic sex ignorance.

5. Details of menstruation, its duration, loss, and discomfort and the age it started.

6. A woman's fertility may be affected by heredity and closely resemble that of her mother's. Your doctor will want to know the pregnancy and birth histories of her mother, sisters, and even brothers.

Following this general investigation for clues in your backgrounds, your wife generally undergoes a series of physical examinations:

1. A vaginal examination in which a routine test for cancer is made.

2. A check on the physical condition of her interior passages which might affect intercourse.

3. Examination for a blockage of her fallopian tubes commonly caused by disease or inflammation.

4. A test of the endometrium to determine if ovulation has occurred and a routine check for a rare, but possible, tubercular condition.

Up to this point, usually only your wife has been involved in the questioning and examinations in the search for the cause of infertility. Now comes your turn.

1. **The postcoital test:** An examination of cervical mucus is carried out twelve to twenty-two hours after you've had intercourse. This should show if the mucus produced by your wife is such to enable your sperm to live. If the results of this

test prove normal with living sperm, a further test of your sperm probably won't be necessary.

2. **The sperm test:** This test examines the volume of your ejaculation, the number and shape of the spermatozoa, and their motility. If your sperm count is high, the test usually doesn't have to be repeated; if low, additional tests will show if your count is consistently low, or varies from time to time. Don't be embarrassed about taking a sperm test. It's a test of fertility, not your virility or masculinity.

If all the background information and basic examinations listed above fail to reveal the cause of infertility, further and more complicated examinations can be undertaken, usually upon your wife.

Now that we've covered the hows and whys of achieving pregnancy, let's look at the ways of preventing it—through contraception.

Chapter 15

Contraception: The Best Ways to Stop Unwanted Pregnancy

The greatest number of children ever produced by one mother was sixty-nine. Someone was either a fantastic egoist or a real loser. To save you this embarrassment and help you plan a sensibly sized family, you should know the relative effectiveness of the various methods of contraception at your disposal today. They vary considerably. And remember that the over-all effectiveness of a contraceptive device or technique depends not only on how good the method but on how efficiently you use it.

Vasectomy: male sterilization

A vasectomy stops your sperm from reaching the urethra and being ejaculated with your semen. In a relatively simple, fifteen-to-thirty-minute operation, the surgeon makes a small incision in the back of your scrotum and severs your two vas deferens tubes. He has to tie off the cut ends to stop them from rejoining, which they would try to do if given the chance. Sometimes a length of tube is removed or the two ends filled to block the tubes. Your sperm production is unaffected, but as it can't pass up the vas any longer, it breaks down and your body absorbs it.

You may have some short-term swelling and tenderness, but by wearing Y-front underpants you'll relieve much of any strain or discomfort. As you may need a day or two for complete recovery, have the operation done over the weekend so you're ready for work on Monday. After his operation, one TV personality conducted his own talk show that evening. Some men resume sexual relations after several days; most within a month.

Its effectiveness: Vasectomy represents one of the most effective forms of contraception, depending upon the skill of your surgeon. There's about a 1 per cent failure rate requiring a second operation. *Warning:* Although no sperm can pass up your vas after the operation, you've previously stored a great deal of it in your ampullar section and it continues to be released into your semen for some time. Your doctor will insist upon a sperm count two to three months after the vasectomy and a second count several weeks later to make sure your semen shows absolutely free of sperm. Until you get his okay, use conventional contraceptive precautions during intercourse.

The major drawback of vasectomy is its irreversibility. The chance of successfully restoring your fertility may be a little less than fifty-fifty. So do a lot of careful thinking before you decide upon this operation. Many surgeons will only perform it for well-adjusted, happy couples who have reached agreement over its need. They won't do it for the convenience of any of you foot-loose, Don Juan bachelors.

The "golden tap" experiment in the United States may be the answer to a reversible vasectomy. Here a tiny gold tube with a stainless steel tap connects the severed ends of your vas. When in the "off" position, the tap blocks the flow of sperm through the vas. Should you later wish more children, you simply have the surgeon re-enter your scrotum to turn the tap "on." If the golden tap proves successful, future refinements may enable you to turn it on and off magnetically without surgery.

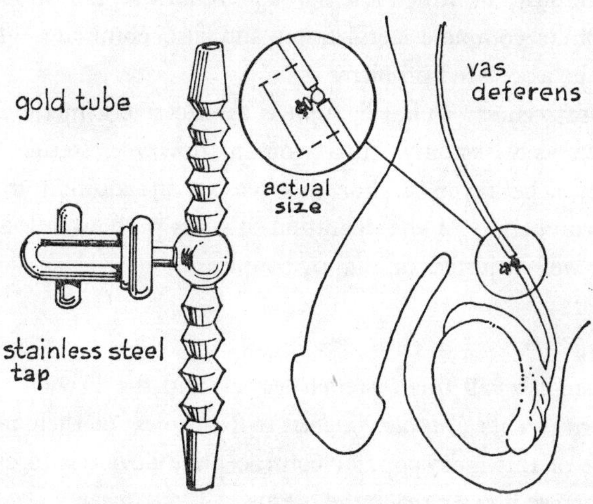

Vasectomy's effect on your virility appears nonexistent. Unless you develop some psychological hang-up, your virility and masculinity shouldn't be affected, and your semen looks unchanged. The major difference lies in your new sexual freedom. A recent survey showed that practically every man enjoyed sex as much or more after the operation. It's been performed on ministers, TV stars, athletes, and ditchdiggers, so no matter what your social and economic group, you're in good company. Over two million men have already had it done in the United States.

Tubal ligation: female sterilization

This operation stops the ova from passing from the ovaries to the uterus. The surgeon cuts the fallopian tubes and ties them off.

There's a great deal of variation in the technique used, but the objective is the same—obstruct the tubes. Ovulation and menstruation continue unchanged, but the tiny unfertilized ova, unable to pass through the fallopian tubes, lose themselves harmlessly among the other organs of the body.

Although not recommended as purely a method of contraception, a hysterectomy, in which the surgeon removes part or all of the uterus, offers complete sterilization and also eliminates menstruation and its associated problems.

Its effectiveness: Tubal ligation is as effective a method of contraception as vasectomy. In a woman, however, sterilization can hardly ever be reversed. For this reason, in addition to the increased complexity of the operation, it's less preferable than vasectomy for well-adjusted and happy couples.

Condoms

The English call them French letters, and the French call them English overcoats (*capote anglaise*). Regardless of their name, the objective of this most popular contraceptive device is to catch and hold semen so it can't reach the uterus.

Using a condom effectively: You can buy condoms in many shapes and varieties; just look in your local "sex shop." Most are long, thin sheaths of latex rubber which you unroll over your erect penis. Condoms in Britain usually have a teat at the tip to hold semen, but Americans seem to prefer a plain tip. In addition to the teat, some brands have a larger bulb to fit more comfortably around your glans while others come lubricated with a slippery silicon compound. The celebrated "ticklers" give erotic stimulation to the vagina with their wild and colorful bumps and tenticles. Thicker latex, reusable sheaths can be purchased, but you've got the cumbersome chore of washing, drying, powdering, and rerolling them. *Warning:* The short American or Grecian tip condom which covers only the glans has been strongly condemned by many experts as unsafe.

When putting on a plain-tipped condom, gently squeeze the tip to form an empty space about half an inch long to hold your ejaculation. This reduces pressure on the rubber. When using a teated condom, make sure you've expelled all the air from the teat before rolling it over your penis.

How effective are condoms? Thanks to modern manufacturing and testing practices, condoms seldom leak or burst during intercourse. The main problem lies in your carelessness. Rough handling can tear or puncture them, completely destroying their purpose. Occasionally men fail to withdraw before losing their erections, so semen may leak around the sides of the sheath. During withdrawal, squeeze the open end of the condom firmly against the base of your penis.

In cases where pregnancy would present a very major problem for those concerned, use a chemical spermicide in addition to your condom. Some brands come prepacked with spermicides which also act as lubricants.

The pill

This female oral contraceptive inhibits ovulation and/or fertilization and implantation of the ova. As such, it's extremely effective in stopping unwanted pregnancy. More than twenty million women throughout the world are estimated to be on the pill today.

Doctors can prescribe three basic types of contraceptive pill, depending upon their patient's reactions to the various formulations.

> **The "combined" pill** is virtually 100 per cent effective and contains both estrogen and progestogen hormones to inhibit ovulation and also create a bad environment for any ova in the uterus and fallopian tubes. Women usually take the combined pill daily for three weeks followed by about seven days of abstention.
>
> **The "sequential" pill** is less effective but still very reliable. Usually a woman takes an estrogen pill for about two weeks and a combined estrogen/progestogen pill for the next week,

followed by a week of abstention. Although it inhibits ovulation, it doesn't produce such a bad environment for fertilization and implantation as the combined pill, and so there's a slightly greater risk of pregnancy should the woman forget to take one of the pills.

The "continuous" pill is the least effective of the three, although more reliable than many other forms of contraception. Women generally take a pill containing progestogen every day. While available in Britain, at the date of writing, the U. S. Food and Drug Administration had not yet given its unqualified approval of this type of pill.

The disadvantages: Aside from the nuisance of remembering when to take the pills, the major disadvantage is the differing reactions of women to the hormonal changes the pills make in their bodies. Some develop side effects of depression, headache, and weight gain. Others often feel happier and healthier and may even find an improvement in their acne and scalp conditions. Current investigations of more dramatic medical complications have been undertaken by teams on both sides of the Atlantic. For this reason, the pill must be prescribed by a doctor who knows his patient's condition and can follow any changes in it.

The male pill

No, it's not here yet, but work continues on the development of a male oral contraceptive. To date, none have been found that don't have some very weird and unpleasant side effects.

Intrauterine devices

No one appears to know exactly why the I.U.D. achieves such a relatively high degree of protection against pregnancy, but it does. These small metal or plastic devices must be fitted within the uterus by a doctor and remain there indefinitely unless dislodged accidentally or withdrawn purposefully. As it has no effect on ovulation, some believe the device affects the motility of your sperm or creates a bad environment in the uterus for ova development. The variety of imaginative designs (I've seen sixteen) indicates the uncertainty over the cause and effect of the I.U.D.s.

Diaphragm and cervical caps

These temporary devices act as barriers to help stop sperm from getting up the cervical canal into the uterus. They should be used with chemical spermicides to increase their effectiveness.

The diaphragm, or "Dutch cap," is a thin rubber dome which women insert over their cervix. The rim contains a flat metal or coil spring to press it firmly against the vagina walls. It comes in various sizes and should be fitted initially by a doctor, after which the woman can insert and remove it at will. Cervical caps and vault caps perform the same basic function and are used in the same way.

Diaphragms and caps should be covered with a spermicide and can be inserted over the cervix up to six hours before intercourse. More spermicide cream, foam, or a suppository must be used if intercourse occurs later than this or is done repeatedly. The cap should be left in for at least six hours after sex to help stop any live sperm from getting up the cervical canal.

Chemical spermicides

These chemicals represent relatively poor contraceptive protection when used alone. They kill sperm in the vagina and, in the case of foam, also act as a barrier against sperm movement into the cervix. The three basic forms are:

> **Creams, gels,** and **pastes,** which should be spread on diaphragms and caps and used to supplement condoms. Insert them into the vagina before and between intercourse.
>
> **Suppositories,** which should be placed in the vagina at least fifteen minutes before sex so they have time to melt, and **foaming tablets,** which are inserted just before intercourse.
>
> **Aerosol foams** are introduced into the vagina by a plunger-type applicator like that used for gels and pastes.

The rhythm method

This relatively ineffective form of contraception relies upon avoiding intercourse during a woman's time of fertility. Your wife must keep track of her approximate time of ovulation based upon the timing of her menstrual cycle. It's more complicated than it seems because her cycle usually varies from month to month and may run anywhere from twenty to forty days.

Here's a typical twenty-eight-day cycle indicating the possible days of fertility and those days "safe" for intercourse:

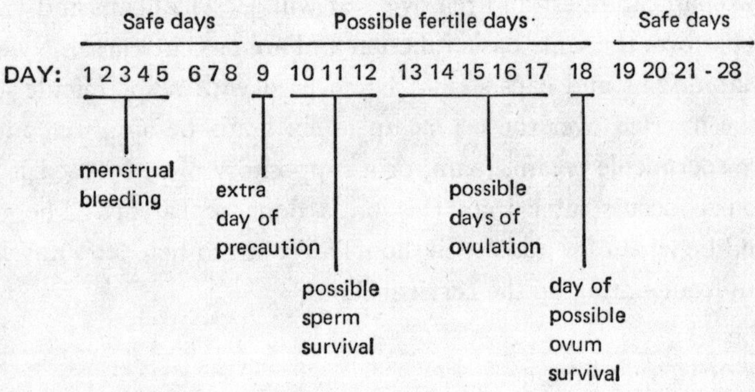

Temperature method

The temperature method represents a more accurate way for a woman to determine her peak fertility times than relying on the calendar start and finish of menstruation, particularly if she has very irregular cycles.

During and just after her period, a woman's temperature remains fairly constant and low. It suddenly shoots up about 2.43 degrees Fahrenheit around the time of ovulation and keeps up until just before the start of her next period. By charting her temperature changes, she can fairly accurately predict her safe days for intercourse. Unfortunately, obtaining accurate temperature readings may be difficult for some women, and both this and the rhythm method require sexual abstinence for ten days or more a month, which many men find unacceptable.

Withdrawal, or coitus interruptus

As its Latin name suggests, this form of contraception has been around for a very long time. It depends upon your being able to withdraw from your woman just before ejaculation. It ranks relatively low for reliability (although not as low as one might think) and takes concentration and considerable willpower. Aside from this drawback, coitus interruptus can be psychologically harmful to establishing a successful and rewarding sexual relationship between two people. Doctors seldom recommend it.

The douching myth

Abandon the practice of flushing semen from the vagina with a douche as a means of contraception. It just doesn't work. Within ninety seconds after a climax, sperm may be out of the vagina and into the cervical canal where no cleansing liquid can reach it. Few women can manage this operation in the time required—even if they're Olympic sprinters. Douching isn't even recommended very often for hygiene purposes because it washes out natural and healthy vaginal secretions. In some emerging nations, a shaken cola bottle often substitutes for a douche. Better to drink it than waste it in this way.

YOUR BEST CONTRACEPTIVE METHOD

To summarize, the over-all effectiveness of a contraceptive device or technique depends upon its inherent effectiveness and how well you use it. A device that may be best for one couple because of their skill in handling it may be the most ineffective one for you.

Bearing this in mind, there's general agreement upon the relative effectiveness of various contraceptive methods in terms of the approximate number of women out of one hundred couples who may become pregnant in one year. This assumes that each method of contraception is used carefully. The high figure for the rhythm method is typical if the method is self-taught and haphazardly used, which in too many cases it is.

Contraceptive Method	*Number of Unwanted Pregnancies Among 100 Women over One Year*
Vasectomy	virtually none
Tubal ligation	virtually none
Combined pill	.7
Sequential pill	1.4
Continuous pill	1–4
Temperature method	.8–1.4
Condoms	2–3
Intrauterine devices	2–4
Diaphragms and caps with spermicides	2–5
Temperature and rhythm methods combined	3.2–8
Spermicides alone	5–18
Withdrawal	5 or more
Rhythm Method	5–40
No contraceptive method	about 40

CHAPTER 16

Venereal Disease: How to Protect Yourself Against It

Recently at dinner, I received quite a surprise from seven highly intelligent and urbane men and women: my mad Portuguese hostess, a striking Egyptian beauty, a flame-haired English divorcée, an Italian fashion model, and their wealthy and successful escorts. The subject of VD came up, and the stories and myths that floated around the table would have been laughable had they not pointed up the basic problem of contracting a serious venereal infection: ignorance. With the exception of our Egyptian beauty who had recently had a blood test, most of these charming people might have had one of the many venereal diseases without even knowing it.

Would you know what to look for? Every man should, and that's why I've included this chapter in the book.

WHO GETS VD?

VD respects only celibacy. If you're at all adventurous sexually, as Kinsey reports so many of us to be, you stand a very good chance of picking up VD and, through ignorance, passing it on. I've known two men who've infected their innocent wives with gonorrhea much to their embarrassment.

Today gonorrhea spreads throughout the world in epidemic proportions, and syphilis kills more people than all infectious diseases combined (excluding tuberculosis). You can't blame the spread on public lavatories and drinking glasses; ninety-nine out of a hundred cases of VD comes from sexual contact.

SYPHILIS: THE KILLER

A poem written in 1530 by a Veronese physician/poet tells of a young swineherd named Syphilis who incurred the wrath of Apollo in the form of a terrible disease. He really mucked things up for us. Syphilis is by far the most serious and deadly of the venereal infections. It strikes men harder than women.

Syphilis comes from a germ (*Treponema pallidum*) which enters your body usually during sexual intercourse through minor defects or abrasions in the skin and mucous membrane. These abrasions can be caused during the act of intercourse itself. The germs can live only a few hours outside the body. They need moisture and body warmth to survive and so thrive in your genital areas, rectum, anus, and mouth. Thus occasionally you can become infected through prolonged contact such as kissing or heavy petting where the genitals touch, but there's no penetration.

Camels can also carry syphilis and transmit it to humans by their bite. A camel bite may represent a valid but rather far-fetched excuse to give your wife unless your business frequently takes you to North Africa.

How long is the incubation period?

The time from infection to the appearance of the first symptoms can range from nine to ninety days, depending upon your natural resistance and immunity to the infection and the virulence of the disease in the person from whom you contracted it. The average incubation period runs between three and four weeks. The germs multiply by simple division every thirty hours. The effects of this reproduction rate are staggering. When the first symptoms appear, the number of treponemes in your body could be in the neighborhood of ten billion.

Symptoms: the three stages of syphilis

The primary stage—look for a chancre:

The primary stage usually begins about three weeks after infection with the formation of a sore or chancre at the place where the treponemes entered your body. In 95 per cent of the cases the sore appears on your penis or genital area: at other times on lips, tongue, in the mouth, rectum, or around the anus.

The chancre usually starts as an oval ulcer which develops into a hard flat buttonlike swelling with a moist central ulcer from which a clear watery liquid oozes. It measures from less than a quarter inch to about a half inch. The chancre is painless and doesn't itch or bleed. When rolled between your thumb and finger, the underlying tissue feels hard, like a small buried pearl. Usually only one chancre appears, but there may be more.

Because of their painless and transient nature, primary chancres often go undetected or ignored. If not treated, they usually heal completely within days or weeks. Some may take up to three months.

Lymph glands about the chancre enlarge noticeably, particularly in the groin. They may be the first symptom of the disease which comes to your attention.

Diagnosis: Doctors treat all genital ulcers as syphilitic until proved otherwise, because the appearance of the chancre occasionally varies from the normal. The presence of syphilis at this stage can be confirmed by a microscopic examination for treponemes in serum obtained from the chancre and less frequently from the juice of lymph glands. Doctors usually take blood tests at weekly intervals for a month and then monthly for the next three months because in the early days all blood tests show negative, not showing positive until five to ten weeks after the initial infection.

The secondary stage—look for the rash

The secondary stage is the most acute and infectious period. The disease has temporarily broken through the body's defense mechanisms and spread throughout your body and its organs where the treponemes continue to multiply. If not treated, this stage will last in varying degrees of intensity for up to four or five years.

A rash usually covering your body, face, and limbs is the most typical symptom. It may vary widely from one person to the next and so can be misdiagnosed. The characteristics common to syphilis rashes are no itching and a tendency to symmetrical distribution. The spots look a dusty red in color, although they may be fainter or more obviously colored.

Other symptoms include superficial skin ulcers, which often appear on the linings of your mouth, throat, genitals, and rectum. They're not painful, but are highly infectious. Loss of voice may result from the formation of one of these ulcers on the larynx, which was why young men in the late nineteenth century were warned to avoid beautiful women with husky voices.

The lymph glands in your groin, under the arms and chin, and on your neck often become enlarged. You may feel tired and feverish, suffer loss of appetite, have headaches and pains in your bones and joints. Bald patches frequently appear if your scalp has been infected, and sometimes your eyes become inflamed. Hepatitis and jaundice may accompany it.

Diagnosis: Treponemes found in the liquid of the superficial ulcers or the discovery of antibodies against the germ in your blood confirms the presence of syphilis. Because your body has had ample time to manufacture these defensive antibodies, blood tests always show positive in this stage.

A problem arises when, through inaccurate diagnosis and treatment, you may have taken antibiotics internally or externally. This reduces the number of treponemes in your bloodstream and on the surface of the skin and so may mask the disease. If this is the case, you must take blood tests over a long period of time.

Because, in some cases, the symptoms of syphilis at this state may be relatively mild and transitory, they can be easily misdiagnosed and the disease may pass untreated to its third stage.

The tertiary stage—Where will it strike?

The tertiary stage shows no outward signs of the disease. The treponemes, now thoroughly entrenched, have reached an uneasy balance within your body. You may be infectious in the first years; however, as the syphilis wears on, you become less likely to infect others. This latent stage can last for months, years, or a lifetime, but at any time the balance may be overcome enabling the disease to attack any part of your body at whim.

Diagnosis: In the absence of external symptoms, syphilis must be diagnosed through positive blood tests, examinations of the cerebrospinal fluid, and X rays of your heart and blood vessels.

WHAT ARE THE EFFECTS OF SYPHILIS?

Based upon existing medical knowledge, between 30 and 50 per cent of men with untreated syphilis will suffer serious, sometimes fatal, physical or mental problems brought on by the disease. The most frequent area of attack involves skin ulceration, the bones, heart and aorta, and your nervous system. It can make your bones and joints very painful, and so damage and weaken the valves of your heart and walls of the aorta that irreversible heart failure occurs. Attacks on the central nervous system affecting the brain and spinal cord can result in mental and physical deterioration leading, in the extreme, to complete insanity and paralysis.

The execution of 3 per cent of the population of England during the reign of Henry VIII may have been related to syphilis of his brain. Many believe Beethoven's deafness was caused by cerebral syphilis, and it is said that Schumann died of it in a mental hospital. Nietzsche, Baudelaire, and other French writers had general paralysis of the insane. Molière died of heart trouble caused by syphilis. This disease doesn't belong just to the history books. Several months ago on a plane to Minorca, a friend confided to me that his college classmate died of syphilis only a few months earlier at the age of forty-two.

Curing syphilis

The best treatment for syphilis is the introducing of penicillin or, in the case of allergy, several other antibiotics into your bloodstream and tissues in a constant and adequate concentration for seven to twenty-one days. The use of long-acting preparations of penicillin have reduced the number of injections needed to maintain this constant antibiotic level, and further research may make only one or two injections necessary.

This treatment effectively cures 90 to 95 per cent of the cases of primary and secondary stage syphilis. The earlier the treatment, the greater your chance for complete recovery. In tertiary syphilis, treatment will usually stop the advance of the infection, but **penicillin cannot restore the damage** done to your heart, nerve tissue, and other organs of your body.

Six to twelve hours after the first injection, about half of the patients with early syphilis (a quarter of those with late syphilis) experience a harmless reaction of fever, sweating, and a headachey feeling, similar to an attack of flu.

Regular blood tests and physical examinations should be carried out for a period of two years after treatment. This surveillance will pick up any relapses or new reinfections. Those in the tertiary stage should be kept under watch for many years and some for the rest of their lives.

DID COLUMBUS START SYPHILIS IN EUROPE?

Two conflicting schools of thought exist over the origin of syphilis. The **Columbian** or New World Theory rests upon the fact that prior to 1492 syphilis was unknown in Europe; no documented descriptions of it existed and none of its effects were uncovered in human bones before the end of the fifteenth century. In 1492 Columbus landed in the West Indies and returned to Spain the following year. Upon the return voyage, many of the crew, who had obviously availed themselves of the delights ashore, showed symptoms of a strange new disease they called Indian measles. A physician in Barcelona reported treating numbers of Columbus' crew for this new illness.

Soon after this, in 1495, Charles VIII of France set siege to Naples using mercenaries from all over Europe. Spanish soldiers enlisted in both the attacking and defending armies, and soon the new disease swept through both sides of the conflict, so weakening the French Army that Charles withdrew and sent his mercenaries home. Their homeward paths are easy to follow. According to records, the infection reached Paris in 1496, London in 1497, and Edinburgh in 1498. Vasco da Gama and his Portuguese crew carried it to India in 1498, and China later reported it in 1505. The English called it the French disease, who called it the Italian disease, who called it . . . and so on around the world.

The **Unitarian** Theory states that the many treponemal diseases like syphilis are different manifestations of a single disease which started millions of years ago with primitive man in Africa.

GONORRHEA

The joke "Here today, gonorrhea tomorrow" is more factual than most of us would like to believe. More than one million Americans contract gonorrhea every year. Although symptoms are usually very apparent in men, doctors have no reliable serum test to confirm the disease in often asymptomatic women. Over half of the women infected with gonorrhea don't know they have it for some time and so act as reservoirs for the infection, carrying it from one man to the next.

Gonorrhea is caused by germs called gonococci which spread on and under the surface of the cells lining your genitals, rectum, and occasionally your throat (pharynx) to set up an inflammation that leads to the production of pus. You almost always pick up these germs through sexual intercourse and anal and oral-genital contact.

How long is the incubation period?

The incubation period commonly takes two to ten days, the average being two to five days after infection. The periods may be as long as thirty days in women and can go unnoticed for a long period of time.

Symptoms of gonorrhea

First you notice an uncomfortable tingling inside your penis, followed at the end of the incubation period by a thick yellow-green discharge. The discharge may vary in viscosity and quantity from man to man, but can generally be found in the morning before passing urine. You usually have a burning sensation while urinating and have the urge to do so more often than normal. (Fourteenth-century England called it the burnings and later intellectuals dubbed it *la chaude pis*). As the infection spreads, your discharge increases, staining underwear, pajamas, and bed linen.

If not treated at this early stage, gonorrhea spreads back along the urethra causing more pain while urinating, and a little blood may be found in the last drops of urine.

Anal symptoms

During anal intercourse gonorrhea is often introduced into the lining of the rectum. There may be no apparent symptoms of discharge and the infected person becomes a carrier of the disease. In this case, the first warning often occurs when the sex partner develops the more tell-tale symptoms in his penis.

Oral symptoms

Infection of your throat (pharynx) generally occurs through oral-genital sex. Symptoms of this infection occur infrequently and can be confused with other, more common throat illnesses. When present, symptoms are varying degrees of discomfort or soreness of your pharynx, abnormal redness of its skin, and discharge.

Possible effects of gonorrhea

Fortunately, gonorrhea is much less dangerous than syphilis, but it has some nasty effects. If neglected for ten to fourteen days, the infection can become severe leading to a contraction of your urethra, making it difficult to pass urine, and to chronic inflammation of your prostate gland. It can also cause a blockage of the tubes carrying sperm, which results in decreased fertility or permanent sterility.

The treatment for gonorrhea

Penicillin or tetracycline taken by injection or orally are the most common and effective treatments for this infection. A 90 per cent cure rate can be expected from an initial regimen of these drugs given at the proper dosage levels.

Exclude alcohol from your diet because evidence shows it increases the chance of relapse. It also reduces inhibitions, which encourages sexual activity during treatment and thereby increases your chances of reinfection or transmitting the disease to others. For obvious reasons, forget sex until your cure is certain. During the weeks following treatment your doctor will probably carry out examinations to make sure you have a permanent cure.

Various strains of gonococci causing this infection don't give up easily, and more and more develop increased resistance to treatment. New, highly resistant strains came home with the troops from Vietnam. In light of the speed with which gonorrhea spreads, this poses a serious threat. Some strains can now be destroyed only with very high doses of penicillin. This makes it even more important for you to seek treatment as soon as possible after the first symptoms appear, before the gonococci establish too strong a foothold.

NONSPECIFIC URETHRITIS

Many nonspecific genital infections, diagnosed as gonorrhea thirty years ago, have become an increasing problem today, particularly in the more affluent areas of the world with the highest standards of personal hygiene. Their cause, infective agent or germ, is not known, and because these diseases cause inflammation of the genital tracts, many victims jump to the conclusion they have gonorrhea. Nonspecific urethritis is the most common condition in this group. It usually attacks men and is generally considered to result from intercourse.

Its incubation period

Symptoms usually appear from seven to twenty-eight days after sex, although the disease may remain latent and unnoticed for much longer periods of time. This represents one of the main points of difference between "N.S.U." and gonorrhea.

What are the symptoms of nonspecific urethritis?

Generally the first symptom appears as a discharge from your penis, usually accompanied by a burning sensation when passing urine. Like gonorrhea, you have the desire to urinate more often.

In the early stages the infection confines itself to the end of your urethra, but if untreated, spreads farther back where either it can cause greater pain or the symptoms lessen.

What are its effects?

This infection can attack your bladder, resulting in more frequent and painful urination and some blood in your urine. It may also invade your testicles causing swelling, pain, and possible sterility.

The disease can develop into an arthritic condition (called Reiter's disease) in about 3 per cent of the infected men and bring pain to the bone joints and inflame your eyes. Sometimes ulcers develop on your mouth and penis.

Treating nonspecific urethritis

Because the cause of this condition remains undetected, the treatment is difficult and not always satisfactory. Antibiotic tablets taken over a period of time or a combination of sulfur formulated tablets and antibiotic injections appear to give the most effective results. These treatments cure about 70 per cent of the cases. For those not helped, doctors use a variety of other antibiotic routes.

As with gonorrhea, give up all alcohol and sex for at least two weeks. To make sure you have been completely cured of this evasive disease, have your doctor make the necessary follow-up examinations.

TRICHOMONIASIS: THE HONEYMOON DISEASE

A minute, one-celled parasite called *Trichomonas vaginalis* (T.V.), found only in the human genital track, causes this very common sexually transmitted condition. Men are the common carriers of T.V.

Honeymoon vaginitis usually happens when the unknowing and infected groom passes on the T.V. to his new bride. After the incubation period, often while still honeymooning, it may become too painful for the bride to engage in intercourse. Many early marital rows start over this.

WHAT ARE THE SYMPTOMS OF T.V.?

Men usually don't have noticeable symptoms because they wash out most of the T.V. parasites clinging to the slippery walls of their urethra every time they urinate. However, parasites can be found under their foreskin. Some men may notice a slight itching or discomfort inside their penis and may experience a little discharge in the morning. Complications from T.V. are rare in men.

Women, on the other hand, offer a secure breeding ground for the parasite, which can live in their vagina for years. Although the incubation period runs between four and twenty-eight days, women may have no symptoms for a long while, or may be hard hit with a large vaginal discharge, itching, and pain.

If your girl friend has a diagnosed condition of T.V., you probably have it, too, even though you have no symptoms. As this condition often accompanies other venereal diseases, it warns you to look for symptoms of more serious infections.

THE CURE IS EASY

Tablets taken orally for one week will cure 80 per cent of the cases. An additional week of treatment usually cures the rest. Again, rule out sex until the T.V. parasite has been destroyed.

CANDIDA

Candida albicans is a fungus commonly found on the skin and sometimes in the vagina of women. It has no apparent symptoms in women.

Possible symptoms

Certain circumstances infrequently cause the fungus to irritate the male genitals. There may be irritation of the tip of your penis and foreskin, and occasionally a discharge. Sometimes men notice an itching and soreness in their penis just after having sex with infected women, and some may develop a skin rash due to their hypersensitivity to the fungus.

A simple cure

The application of antibiotic ointments to your skin cures this condition. Symptoms usually disappear within a few days.

VIRAL WARTS

Two viral infections, warts and herpes, were discussed in Chapter 3, but should be mentioned here.

Viral warts are infectious and can be spread from one person to another through sexual contact. Genital warts occur on the skin and mucous lining of the genitalia. On the skin, the warts are horny. On the mucous surfaces they appear more papular, like small tumors. Warts on the hand can be spread to your genitalia by touching or scratching them. Warts behave in an unpredictable way and may vanish of their own accord or require one of several treatments for removal.

HERPES

The herpes virus can cause inflammation and blistering of the skin of your penis. Not only can sexual intercourse activate it, but this infectious virus can be transmitted during sexual contact to your lips and genital areas.

SCABIES

Beware of the things that crawl in the night. *Sarcoptes scabiei* is a round, eight-legged parasite barely visible to the naked eye which moves from one body to another during periods of intimate contact such as sharing the same bed.

The female burrows under the horny skin surface to lay her eggs. This condition usually occurs between your fingers, on the wrists, genitals, and buttocks. A secondary eruption of papules, often scattered over your body and limbs, results from your skin's allergic reaction to the scabies. These eruptions itch, and your scratching can lead to scabbing and secondary infections. The incubation period is four to six weeks, because itching occurs only after your skin becomes sensitive to these creatures.

Treating scabies

You treat this condition by applying an emulsion all over the body for two consecutive days. On the day following each application, scrub your skin with soap and hot water.

CRAB LICE

These lice, which the French call butterflies of love (*papillons d'amour*), spread during intimate contact. They are visible as tiny gray dots and generally cling to the roots of pubic hair, although in severe infestations they attach themselves to body hair—even eyebrows and head hair. The eggs, or nits, fasten firmly to the hair and aren't easily detached.

Symptoms

These creatures make you itch but produce no other symptoms such as a rash. For this reason, crab lice may establish a flourishing colony before coming to your attention, especially if you haven't been host to them before.

Treating crabs

Destroy the lice by applying insecticide powders and lotions which you get from your pharmacist. Take care to rid yourself of the nits; this might require a second application ten days or so later. The usage instructions vary depending upon the type of preparation used for the treatment. Your clothes, bed linens, and towels should be laundered in hot water or dry-cleaned.

A person who passes on lice may be careless about the treatment of VD. Crab lice and scabies often accompany other venereal diseases, particularly gonorrhea, and so while treating them, look for possible symptoms of other venereal infections.

PRECAUTIONS TO TAKE AGAINST VD

A combination of factors, each magnifying the other, makes it obvious why VD has reached epidemic proportions today. Over the last decade or so, freer morality has lead to more premarital intercourse and an increase in promiscuity. Girls mature and enter into sexual activities at an earlier age without the sophistication and knowledge of a more experienced person. The VD rate among teen-age girls is far higher than that for any other age group.

The role of the prostitute as a disease spreader has been usurped by promiscuous amateurs, the girls who have jobs, live away from home, and enjoy sexual relationships with more than one man, particularly when inhibitions have been lowered by a few drinks at a party. Add to this the fact that so many women are undetected reservoirs of VD, plus the increasing resistance to treatment of many infectious strains, and it becomes obvious why you should take some precautions if you want to play.

The surest prevention against VD is either celibacy or a faithful sexual relationship with only one person. You more adventurous men must accept the risks, but cut them to the minimum:

1. Use a condom *and* make sure your penis or hands have not come in contact with your partner's sex organs before putting on the sheath.
2. Handle your penis as little as possible after sex.
3. Urinate soon afterward to clean out the urethra, and wash your genital areas with soap and water. These precautions may reduce risk of infection but are certainly far from 100 per cent effective.
4. Depending upon your sex activity, have periodic VD checks with your doctor.

If you've slept with a stranger or someone of whom you're not absolutely sure, keep an eye open for the following symptoms.

a. A tingling in your penis or pain while urinating
b. Discharge from your penis, particularly in the morning
c. Chancres on your penis, genital areas, or lips
d. Rashes
e. Irritation or itching of the genital areas.

If you notice any of these symptoms, consult your doctor or visit a public VD clinic as soon as possible for diagnosis and treatment if needed. Venereal disease should not be considered embarrassing or the sign of being "dirty" or a social outcast.

Inform the person from whom you may have contracted the infection and those with whom you have slept since, so they can take appropriate action.

And remember, you can develop immunity to measles, mumps, and chicken pox, but not to VD.

Chapter 17

Physical Fitness: How to Build a Healthier Body with the Least Effort

To live a young, healthy, and active life, no matter what your age, you've got to *be* fit as well as *look* fit. The purpose of the next three chapters is to make you both, and to do it quickly and efficiently with as little effort as possible.

You've got to face one fact, however: You can't get into shape and stay there without a little work. But it can be done a lot more easily than you may think. For perhaps the first time, you're going to be doing a simple exercise regimen specifically designed to make the most of your body, not someone else's. And to get you in condition even faster, I'll show you how to turn your whole day into one continuous fitness exercise—one you'll hardly know you're doing.

Read these chapters thoughtfully and follow the instructions with care. The more thought you put in at the start, the sooner you'll see results. You've got to understand what fitness is all about and what level of fitness is best for you.

YOUR IDEAL LEVEL OF FITNESS

Every man has his own "ideal" level. Yours is the level at which mind and body most effectively meet all the demands put on them by your life-style, your work, and other activities. Your body has to meet four criteria before you reach your ideal level:

Specific muscle fitness: Each of your muscles should be flexible and strong enough to complete all your normal daily activities without stiffness, pain, or getting overtired. You need a little extra flexibility and reserve strength to cope with any emergency or unusual situation which may crop up.

General fitness: Your internal support systems (your cardiovascular, respiratory, and other systems) should be fit enough to support all your body's daily activities without undue strain and fatigue. They, too, need a little reserve for emergencies.

Posture: Your body should stand or sit in that upright position which enables it to function at peak efficiency and which it can hold with minimum muscle effort. Like the mast of a ship, your body weight should be dispersed evenly down your spine to your feet. Your muscles act like rigging to hold the spine's vertical position against the pull of gravity.

Ego fitness: The attractiveness of your over-all physique is more important to your psychological than your physical well-being and depends, to a great extent, upon what's in vogue and how you want to look. In the 1950s it was beefcake; today it's the Mr. Averages. One or the other, as long as you have a firm body whose parts are all in good proportion with each other and you haven't a bulging stomach or sagging muscles, you've got an attractive body.

THE FOUR RULES FOR FITNESS

The average man's peak fitness years fall between the ages of eighteen and twenty-five, so most of us have an uphill fight to get into proper shape. You can do it most effectively with a simple regimen of daily exercise and activity founded on four basic fitness rules:

Rule 1: Stretch your muscles

Your muscles and cartilages tend to contract during rest and disuse. The problem increases with age, poor posture, and the more sedentary your life. If you don't halt and reverse this process, you'll be letting yourself in for a lot of muscle stiffness and pain later on. Simple as it may sound, all you've got to do is stretch. Animals do it instinctively—why not you? One really good stretch of your muscles in all directions every morning will help keep them toned, flexible, and loose, and your body will move with more grace and confidence.

Rule 2: Strengthen your muscles a bit each day

Strength is simply your ability to exert a force against resistance, whether it's holding up a weight or holding in your stomach. No matter how great your earlier level of strength, you can't possibly retain it without some exercise, particularly if you've got a desk job. Disuse has a direct and reverse effect on muscle strength and size. For example, the muscles of an arm confined to a cast for only ten days will shrink (atrophy) noticeably. Fortunately for you, muscles recover strength very quickly. With only a few weeks of correct training, you should be able to strengthen any disused muscles dramatically. It's not as hard to keep strong as you may think.

RULE 3: EXERCISE YOUR CARDIOVASCULAR SYSTEM

Of perhaps greatest importance to your fitness is your heart. It pumps blood to your muscles to supply them with the oxygen and nutrients they need to fuel their activity. Without an adequate blood supply, they'd exhaust themselves. During periods of extreme activity, a trained athlete's muscles may call for up to sixty times more oxygen than while at rest. That's one hell of an increase. His cardiovascular system meets this demand in three ways: (1) the capillaries of the inactive muscles close while those of the active ones open wide to divert up to five times more blood to the active muscles, (2) these muscles triple the efficiency with which they take oxygen from the blood, and (3) the heart pumps harder and faster to increase its output by as much as four times. To a lesser extent, your cardiovascular system goes through the same drill every time you climb stairs, play tennis, or swim. You've got to keep your system fit enough to bear the strain your activities put on it, or you're in trouble.

RULE 4: STAND TALL

Poor posture throws your torso weight out of balance so each of your vertebrae and the intervertebral disks fall under twisting, shearing, and crushing pressures. When you think these disks become so squashed during the day that you lose half an inch in height, you'll understand the considerable force on them. (Fortunately, they recover at night while you sleep.) Over the years, torture of this magnitude can cause disk damage and considerable pain. Why chance it? Holding good posture doesn't take any real effort, just getting used to it.

Now that you know the rules, let's put together the simplest and most efficient way for you to carry them out.

HOW TO BUILD YOUR PERSONAL FITNESS REGIMEN

First, take a hard, thoughtful look at yourself and compare each part of your body, inside and out, to the criteria for fitness. Are all your muscles as flexible as they should be; can you touch your chin to each shoulder, lean over without any strain? Does your body feel particularly tired after work or sports? If so, which part—your legs, back, neck? Do you breathe heavily and does your heart pound after a little exertion? Do you see bulges around your waist and the beginning of a pot? Give yourself the complete once-over.

Now put together an exercise regimen that will make the most efficient use of your time. List on paper your fitness problems. Then do each of the exercises in Appendix 4 once or twice very slowly with enough effort to feel exactly which muscles they stretch or strengthen. Choose a variety (not too many) which not only exercise your entire body but place special emphasis on correcting your major problems.

When putting together your regimen, bear in mind what other activities you normally do during the day so there's no duplication of effort. If you're a stevedore, there seems little point in doing arm-strengthening exercises at night; lawn tennis champions shouldn't need much cardiovascular exercise except during off season.

Make sure your regimen can be done in no more than ten or fifteen minutes. If you can't do all your exercises in this time, divide them into two groups and do them on alternate days. If you get bored with or don't like one exercise, substitute a more pleasant one which has about the same effect on your body. Distract and amuse yourself while exercising. I look at TV or listen to the news.

Be sure to make the difficulty of your starting regimen compatible with your age, weight, health, and current physical condition. If you're middle age and over, out of condition, or suspect health complications, ask your doctor to review your regimen and find out how much strain you can afford to put on your heart. Too vigorous an effort can hurt you, so be guided by these important don'ts.

Don't do anything that hurts or puts what feels like excessive strain on your muscles or skeletal structure. Work up gradually to different stretch and strengthening exercises.

Don't exhaust yourself; slowly build up the number of repetitions of each exercise as it becomes easier for you to do.

Don't let your heart "pound." A normal pulse rate runs about 70 beats per minute, plus or minus 10. If you're in good health and have been in training for some time, you have to increase your rate to between 120 and 150 to benefit your cardiovascular system. If you're not in condition, go easy until your fitness level improves.

Don't do isometrics unless you're in good health. They can be harmful to men with heart conditions and high blood pressure. Precede them with warm-up isometrics at half force and gradually work up to maximum force.

What about using a gym?

If you decide to go to a gymnasium for professional help, make sure they give you personal treatment designed for the specific needs of your body. Don't let them throw you right into a regimen of class exercises which might put too much or too little strain on your muscles and heart. Unfortunately, too few gyms take the time or have the knowledge to put your body through the right training course. Good ones can do a fantastic job. One in London works hand in glove with the cardiac section of a major hospital to get businessmen with heart conditions back on their feet so they can lead active lives again. Part of this course deals with training the mind. We'll talk more of that later.

HOW TO GET THE MOST OUT OF EACH EXERCISE

Stretching exercises are isotonic contractions involving muscle contractions and extensions which move your joints. Do them slowly in a continuous, flowing movement and extend your limbs as far as possible. Jerky movements will only set up counterproductive reflex muscle action. Five repetitions of pure stretching exercises should be enough.

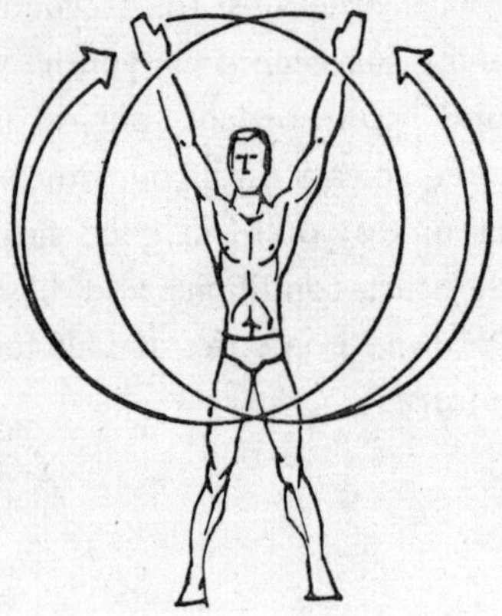

As an example, try the Cross Circle Stretch. Stretch your arms to their limit over your head. Keeping them extended, slowly move them in circles that overlap in front of your chest. You should feel all the muscles of your upper torso pulling.

If your muscles are already contracted from disuse or are in spasm for one reason or another, stretch them gradually with continuous and progressive exercise over a period of time. Only part of the muscle elongation you achieve during each session will be retained to the next.

General fitness isotonics that stimulate your cardiovascular and respiratory systems should be done briskly and in sufficient numbers to make you breathe heavily or pant. Keep increasing the number as they become easier to do. Use these exercises for warming up before sports, because they increase your blood circulation.

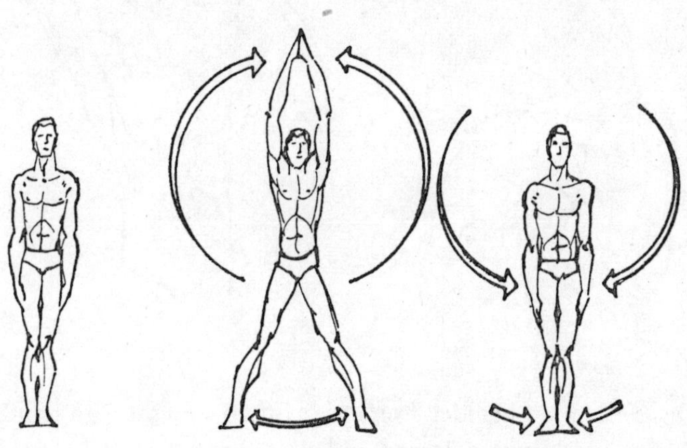

Windmill Jumps are good general fitness exercises. Stand at rest with your hands at your sides. Jump, coming back to rest with your feet apart and your hands together over your head. Jump again, swinging your hands back to your sides, and bring your feet together. Combine these actions in a continuous, flowing movement.

Strengthening exercises involve isometric contractions with little or no joint movement because the contractions are opposed by an equal and opposite force. They effectively strengthen those muscles under tension, but have little effect on your general physical fitness. Hold isometric contractions at maximum force no more than six seconds. Don't do more than two or three repetitions during an exercise session and separate them with a brief rest period. The stomach isometric can usually be held up to a minute at full force if you move the rest of your body while doing it.

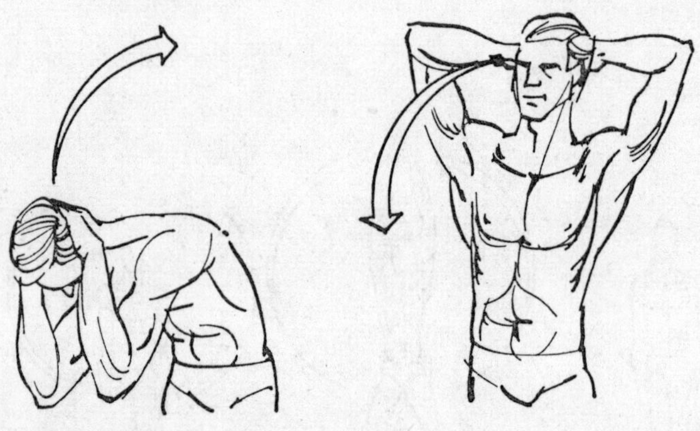

The Neck and Shoulder Isometric: Stand straight with hands behind your head, hands clasped and elbows together. Pull your head down against resistance from your neck. Slowly raise your head to an upright position against strong resistance from your arms. Elbows should gradually open as you raise your head. Keep your back flat and let your chest rise with the action.

Combined isotonic/isometric contractions can be found in many exercises like sit-ups and knee bends. As you would expect, these exercises stretch and strengthen muscles and often build general fitness. Do them slowly and smoothly for maximum benefit and breathe deeply.

The number of times you do each is up to you. A fixed number of repetitions over a period of time will bring you up to a certain level of strength, no further. In health, doubling the number of times you do the exercise will give you some increase in general fitness, but won't double your strength. Rather than doing more than twenty-five repetitions of an isotonic/isometric exercise, you'll increase your muscle strength more by increasing the intensity of the exercise. Either add resistance to your movement by holding weights or substitute a new and more difficult exercise.

THE POSTURE EXERCISES

To have good posture, first you've got to know what it feels like—most men don't. If you think this sounds silly, get up right now and try the Pelvic Tilt exercise. As easy as it looks, I'll bet you can't do it unless you went to military school.

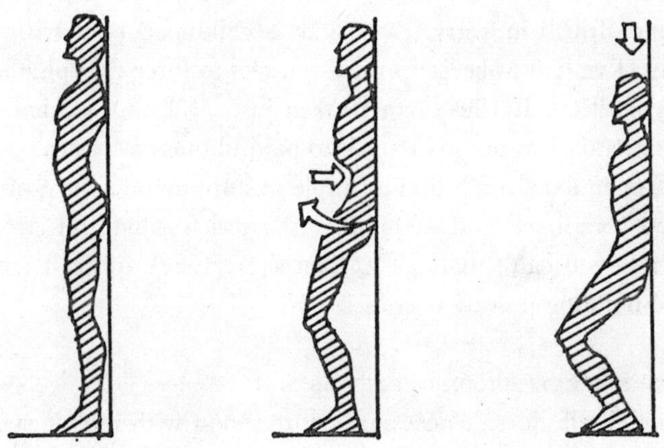

The **Pelvic Tilt** Vertical: Stand with your hands on your hips and your buttocks, shoulders, elbows, and head against the wall. Suck in your stomach and tighten your buttocks while slowly rotating or tilting your pelvis forward until the curve of your lower spine flattens and presses against the wall. Your knees will bend slightly. You may have to use your hands to help tilt your pelvis until you get the hang of it.

After repeating the tilt ten times, hold the position and slowly slide down the wall about eighteen inches and come back up while keeping your lower back, head, shoulders, and elbows pressed to the wall. You'll feel this exercise pulling and flexing your lower back muscles. It forms the basis for many of the posture exercises and can often be used to relieve backache. Now if you move away from the wall, stand as tall as you can, square your shoulders, look straight ahead, suck in your stomach, and tilt your pelvis forward, you'll know what good posture feels like.

To help hold good posture, you've got to strengthen the girdle muscles supporting your spine—your abdominal and back muscles. I can't emphasize enough the importance of this and the potential disability and pain you may face if you neglect it. Backache represents the second or third major cause of lost working hours in American and British industry. Ever since a childhood bout with poliomyelitis, I've had to keep up these muscles to force my spine into its proper position. If I let them weaken just a bit, any sudden movement or strain can put my back into painful muscle spasms.

In Appendix 4 you'll find a simple posture maintenance program to keep your back and abdominal muscles flexible and strong. If physically you can't manage it, then slowly work up to it with the muscle-building posture exercises.

Ego, or muscle-building, exercises

Muscle bulk doesn't necessarily correspond with muscle strength. If your prime objective is to increase muscle bulk, do isotonic contractions against less than maximum resistance. More repetitions of an exercise done against less than maximum loads will build more muscle bulk than fewer repetitions at maximum loads, which builds greater strength. Training with weights builds muscle bulk very quickly, but be careful not to go too far with one muscle group to the exclusion of others or you'll throw your body out of proportion. A rather thin French egoist built himself a massive upper torso, but unfortunately it looked quite ridiculous on top of his neglected "bird" legs. Also, what you build you have to keep up, and that can be a chore.

If you want to add weight to your frame in addition to muscles, review Chapter 11. I recommend against following the route of professional body builders who take injections of male hormones (anabolic steroids) which, when combined with diet and training, can add up to seventy pounds of muscles in only five months. The bulk drops off just as quickly if they don't keep at it. Steroids may also have potentially harmful side effects and should be taken only under medical supervision.

A SAMPLE EXERCISE REGIMEN

Here's the daily regimen of ten exercises that I put together for myself. I've included the entire posture maintenance program, which has the added benefit of keeping my stomach flat. To this I've added only Press-ups to strengthen my upper torso and arms and the Windmill (which I enjoy doing more than running in place) for general fitness. The other exercises (asterisked) I do throughout the day in addition to a lot of muscle stretching to pep up my brain. You'll note that some exercises, like the "U," appear several times because they strengthen or stretch more than just one part of the body.

EXERCISE	PURPOSE		
	Stretch	*Strength*	*General*
Back			
Pelvic Tilt Vertical	x		
The "U"	x	x	some
Leg Roll	x	x	some
Spine Extension No. 2		x	
Forehead to Knees	x		
Abdomen			
The "U"		x	some

Leg Roll		x	some
Abdominal Hold Isometric*		x	
Buttocks			
Pelvic Tilt Vertical		x	
Spine Extension No. 2		x	
Legs			
Pelvic Tilt Vertical		x	
The "U"	x	x	some
Forehead to Knees	x		
Spine Extension No. 2		x	
Neck, Shoulders, Chest, and Arms			
Press-up		x	x
Neck and Shoulder Isometric*	some	x	
Chin Firmer*	x	x	
Cardiovascular			
Windmill			x

This brings us to one of the real secrets of keeping fit.

TURN YOUR WHOLE DAY INTO A FITNESS EXERCISE

Turn everything you do into a form of simple exercise so you effectively double or triple your daily exercise time and effort without really noticing. As a bonus, it will greatly improve your working efficiency.

Stretch throughout the day not only to tone your muscles but to stimulate your nervous system and keep your mind fresh and alert. Do it for a minute or two between meetings and break up long periods of mental concentration to relieve tension. Repeat the drill at night before going to bed to relax yourself.

You can strengthen muscles in ways that may never have occurred to you. For example, don't sit, but stand balanced on one leg while putting on your socks and tying your shoelaces. You'll feel a strong muscle contraction in your legs. When you sit in or get up from a chair or the floor, don't use your hands for support; instead throw all your weight on your leg, abdomen, and back muscles. Suck in your stomach in an isometric contraction as you walk about. For the next few days think about everything you do in these terms.

Some experts recommend thirty minutes of heavy breathing activity every day to keep your cardiovascular system fit. Don't shout "Impossible." It is possible with a little bit of ingenuity.

Walk farther and faster. Park your car farther from the office or get off the bus a stop earlier and walk the rest of the way at a pace brisk enough to make you breathe a bit hard. I usually walk anywhere within a twenty-minute radius, and walk at a clip that many friends find uncomfortable.

Use the stairs. Climb stairs two at a time rather than ride up in the elevator or escalator. I never felt better than when living in a fourth-floor walk-up in Greenwich Village.

Enter into sports. Play squash, tennis, or swim several times a week. Leave the car with your wife and ride a bicycle to work (as many now do in Europe) or to the commuter station. You might end up a healthier one-car family. You'll find lots of activities to include in your daily routine which will make it not only more fun but healthier as well.

TRY THIS "EXECUTIVE SHAPE-UP ROUTINE"

You can do it throughout the day in your office, and the results can be dramatic. A rather plump young assistant of mine did the Abdominal Hold Isometric twice a day for two weeks. His abdominal muscles firmed up so well that his trousers kept falling down. He became the secretaries' delight.

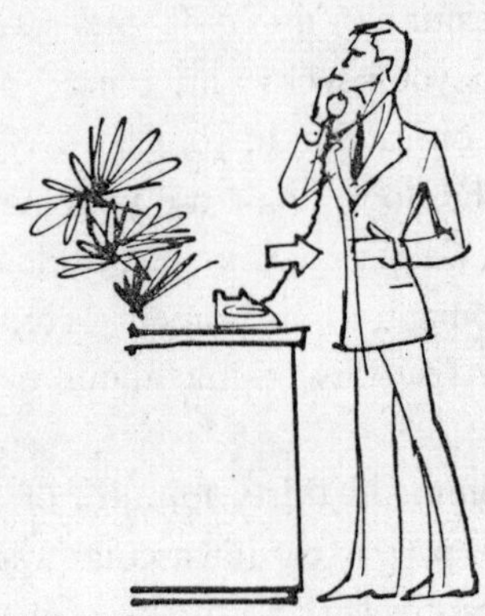

When you answer your phone, suck in your stomach in an isometric contraction and continue to breathe and talk naturally. Hold a maximum force contraction no more than one minute. This will strengthen your abdominal muscles and help flatten your stomach.

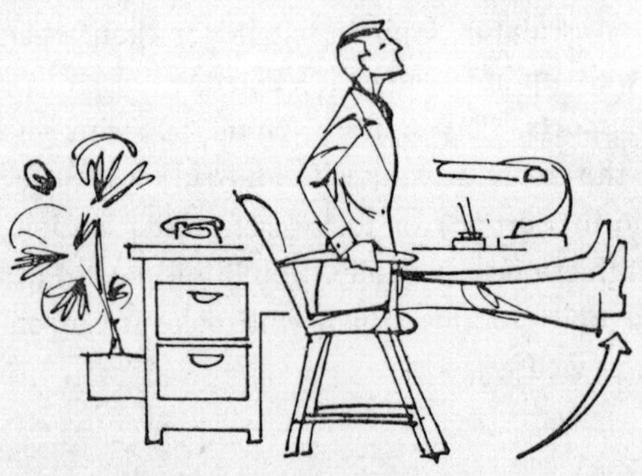

Sit on the edge of a solid, well-balanced chair. Lift your feet as high off the floor as you possibly can while keeping your legs straight. Hold on to the chair for support. Maintain the muscle contraction for six seconds. Repeat it five times throughout the day. This will strengthen your legs, thighs, and abdomen, and stretch your lower back.

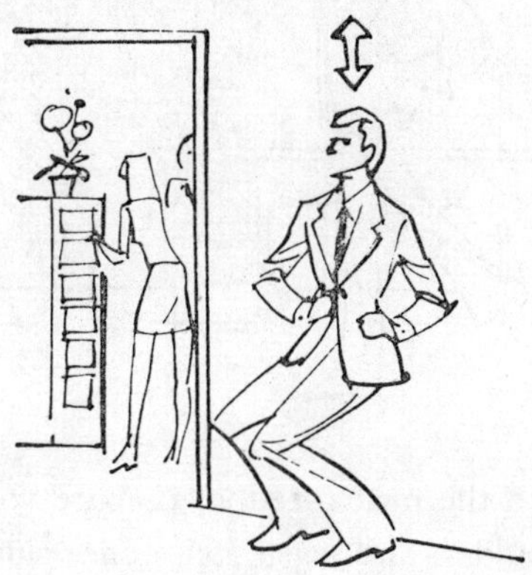

After you've been sitting for some time, do twenty-five Pelvic Tilts (making sure to contract your buttocks) to stretch and ease your lower back muscles. (See page 221.)

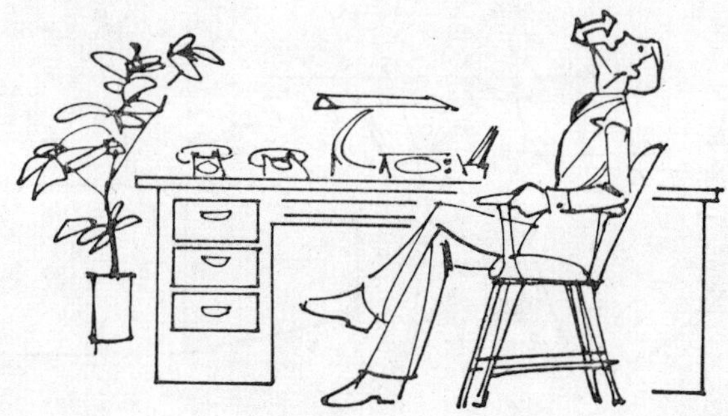

During those rare moments when you get a chance to be alone and think, square your shoulders, tilt your head far back, and do ten chin firming exercises, opening and closing your mouth to firm up the beginnings of the double chin.

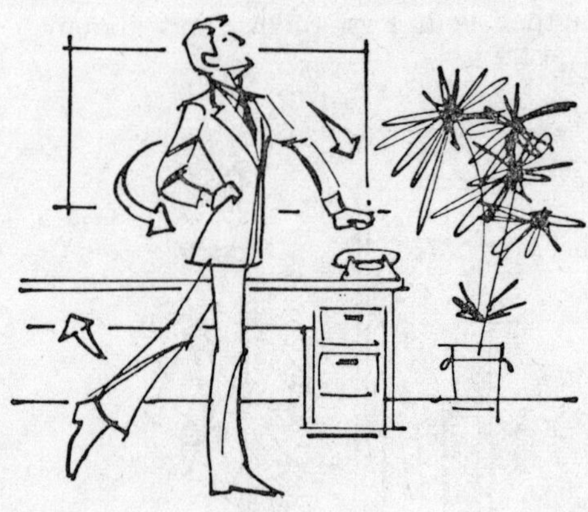

Before going into the next meeting, prepare yourself by stretching your back, shoulder, and leg muscles once slowly to relax your body and freshen up your mental processes.

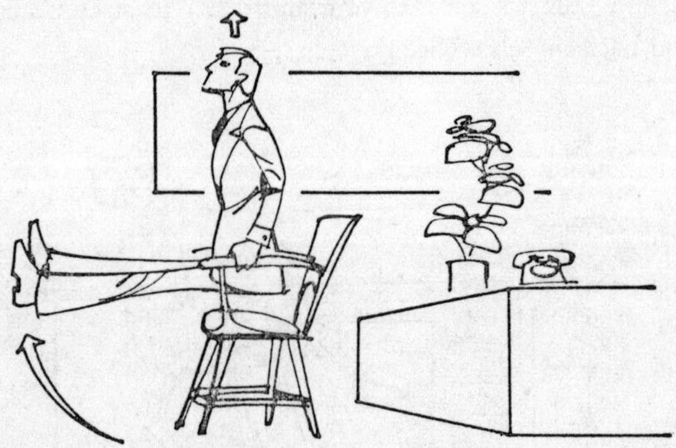

Keeping your legs at right angles to your body, grasp the chair arms and raise and lower your body five times. This will strengthen your arm, shoulder, back, and abdominal muscles. For God's sake, make sure your chair is a stable one or you may propel yourself out a fifty-second-floor window.

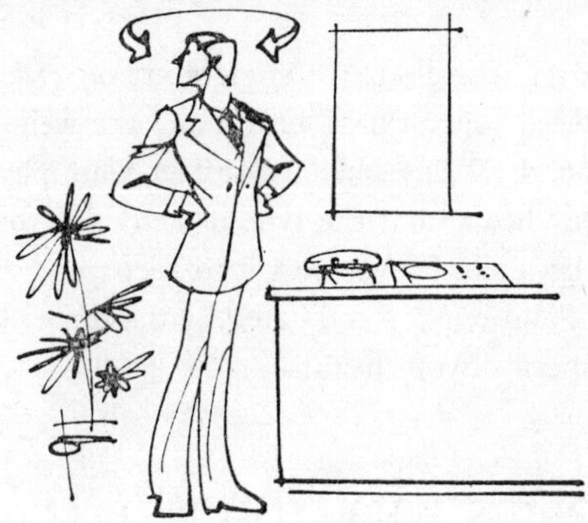

From time to time, rotate your head and look over each shoulder as hard as you can to stretch your neck muscles. Touch your chin to your shoulders. This exercise is also effective in keeping the back stabbers at bay.

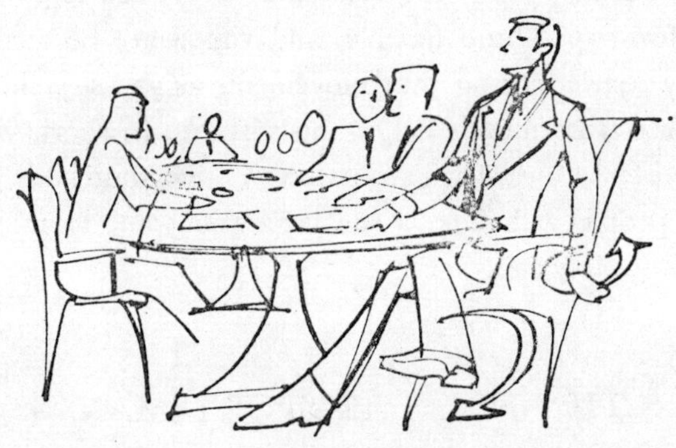

When trapped at a conference table for a long time, cross your legs and slowly swivel one foot after the other to stretch your lower leg muscles and relax your thighs. Try the same thing with your hands and wrists. No one will notice these seemingly common movements.

KEEP YOUR WEIGHT AND HEALTH UNDER CONTROL

Last but not least, your over-all health and the weight your body has to carry around all day obviously affect your physical fitness, the strain on your heart, and the type of activities you can do. If you're going to be really fit, you've got to keep your weight down, get enough sleep, and relax. Read carefully the three chapters dealing with these aspects of your health.

WHEN WILL YOU BE FIT?

You'll instinctively know when you've reached your right level of fitness by what you do and don't feel, and when your doctor slaps you on the back with his congratulations. At the end of a typical day you won't feel too tired for some after-work activities. You'll stop playing tennis, cricket, or swimming, because you're bored with it, not because you're too winded or exhausted to go on. Your body will feel supple and flexible, and you won't be aware of its putting any restrictions on your movements as you stretch or bend. You'll be free from muscle aches and stiffness. In short, when you reach your ideal fitness level, you won't notice your body much at all—other people will. That's the level you want to maintain as long as you possibly can.

TIPS FOR THE SPORTSMAN

Sports afford you a far more enjoyable way of keeping fit than doing exercises, but once a week on Sundays isn't a suitable substitute. Sports strengthen only those muscles that come into play, and so regard them as good for your general fitness, endurance, and muscle flexibility, not as over-all muscle strengtheners. Swimming is a great sport because you have to use almost every muscle in your body to do it well. Golf, aside from getting you out in the fresh air and sunshine, doesn't do much for your general fitness unless the course is hilly enough and you walk fast enough to make yourself pant.

How to increase your endurance with "interval" training

The basis of "interval" training is to expend maximum muscle effort for short periods of time interspersed with brief periods of rest. Today, many coaches consider it better than continuous, unbroken training periods for increasing the effectiveness of your cardiovascular system in meeting the oxygen demands of your muscles. When you jog continuously, your heart falls into a pattern and the strain on it lessens. But interval training surprises your heart and breaks its rhythm so that it has to work harder. That's why only those of you in good physical condition should use it. Swim or run hard for two minutes, then rest for two, then swim, rest, and so on. Start with some warm-up exercises to get your circulation going before really exerting yourself.

Improve your skill to improve your endurance

The best way to get in shape for a sport is to do it. When you train yourself to do something, you force the muscles and support systems of your body to adapt to the specific demands of that sport. This gradually increases the skill and efficiency with which you use your muscles and so reduces their energy requirements. A skilled swimmer may use only one-fifth the energy required by an amateur moving at the same speed.

Once you've developed a skill, it's hard to lose. It's your skill that enables you to put on a pretty good show on the ski slopes or in the swimming pool on the once-a-year vacation. It compensates for your muscle weakness while giving them a chance to regain their strength and flexibility.

How to strengthen individual sporting muscles

Do sporting isometrics. For example, if you hold your tennis racket up in a serving position and press it hard against a wall in that position, you'll create isometric contractions of all the muscles involved in serving and thus strengthen them. Hold the contraction for six seconds, relax, and hold again. Do the same for your forehand and backhand strokes. Use the same technique to strengthen the muscles you use in your golf swing, batting arm, and in other sports.

Easing muscle soreness

General soreness often develops after extreme activity when your muscles haven't yet got rid of all the waste materials created as by-products of their activity. These waste products will be carried off normally by your blood in three to four hours, but you can speed relief by gently exercising to increase your blood circulation.

More serious localized soreness occurring from eight to twenty-four hours after muscle activity may be due to an injury or rupture of your muscle fibers. Rest, heat, and a little *minor* exercise to prevent interfiber adhesion is usually the best cure. Persistent or severe soreness may show more serious underlying problems and you should consult your doctor.

Muscle stiffness and pain

During activity, fluid collects in your muscles causing them to swell and shorten. They thus put up increased resistance to stretching and so give you the feeling of stiffness. Again, after some hours, your bloodstream carries off the fluid, and your muscles can return to their normal length and flexibility.

Muscles can also cause irritation and pain by putting abnormal pressures on the nerves passing between and around their fibers. Surprising as it may seem, this pain helps protect your body from itself. A quick movement or unaccustomed activity which threatens a muscle with damage can cause a jolt of pain. The jolt puts the muscle in a "protective spasm," an involuntary contraction resisting further movement of the offending type. This severe contraction puts painful pressure on the surrounding nerves, which reinforces the contraction long after the initial cause has disappeared.

To relieve this pain, you've got to relax the contracted muscles and so relieve their pressure on the nerves. Use gentle stretching exercises or heat treatment (ultrasound or diathermy treatments give deep, penetration heat). In severe cases, traction may be needed to force muscle stretching. Your coach or doctor will recommend which one or a combination of these treatments best suits your particular problem.

Sports and your sex life

A fit, well-maintained body leads to improved sex, both in frequency and in quality. Sexual intercourse doesn't drain much energy or put much strain on your cardiovascular system—only about the equivalent of climbing a flight of stairs or walking fast for a few seconds.

Contrary to accepted belief, some evidence now shows that sexual activity can be of positive benefit to athletic performance as long as it doesn't interfere with sleep. One Olympic middle-distance runner broke the world record an hour after having intercourse.

WARNING: YOUR BLOOD PRESSURE, THE SAUNA, AND EXERCISE

Your blood vessels are elastic. When you rest, all the vessels in your body remain partially closed to keep the flow of blood under normal pressure. If they were all to relax and open up at the same time, you wouldn't have enough blood to fill the vessel network and your blood pressure would drop dramatically.

The heat in saunas and steam rooms relaxes and dilates your

complete vessel network, resulting in a drop in your blood pressure. Your heart swings into action to restore normal pressure by desperately pumping harder and faster to push more blood into the vessels, but there just isn't enough to fill them. Your pulse rate climbs up and up and so does the strain on your heart.

After five minutes, eight at the most, get out of the sauna and cool off. Unfortunately, men often become so engrossed in conversation while in saunas and steam rooms, they pay little attention to their bodies' urgent signals to escape. If you must go in for this dubious activity, be very careful.

Beware some types of exercise

Your blood pressure increases with exercise. The increase depends on the volume of blood your heart has to pump to fuel your muscle activity and the amount of resistance to it by the vessels. When you use lots of muscles, a large section of your vessel network opens to help the blood reach them. Thus, resistance to circulation is low and the increased blood pressure comes almost entirely from the increased output of your heart.

But when you do exercise that uses only a few small muscle groups (like shoveling snow, which uses primarily your arm muscles), only a few of the vessels open while the rest contract. This greatly increases the resistance to blood being pumped by your heart and results in a more dramatic rise in your blood pressure. If you shovel snow, do some type of warm-up exercise to open your vessel network and so lower your blood pressure.

Chapter 18

Mental Fitness: Standing Up Better Under Stress

One of the best ways of increasing your working effectiveness so you can take on more responsibility is to reduce and adjust to the mental stress and tension in your life. Your mental fitness plays an essential role in your job success and physical survival: far greater than you probably suspect. Stress, tension, and aggression dramatically lower your ability to work, and unless controlled, these mental states can produce changes in your blood pressure and blood chemistry which may lead to heart disease and other illness. Your general fitness and the smooth function of your body rely on the fitness of your mind.

Nature used to have things all worked out so man's mental and physical functions complemented each other, but not now. When a primitive man found himself in a tense situation, like a charging tiger, his body automatically released adrenaline which liberated the fatty acids needed to fuel his muscles for fight or flight. They also made his blood "stickier" so he'd heal faster in case that tiger got its claws into him.

Unfortunately, nature didn't foresee your problem today—that of building up a lot of mental tension and aggression in your business and home which you can't relieve with muscle activity. Without movement, your body doesn't use up those extra fatty acids. They circulate through your blood vessels and may convert into cholesterol which many cardiologists believe lines the arteries to restrict blood circulation and thus put increasing strain on your cardiovascular system. Studies also link tension directly to mental and physical illnesses other than just those of your heart.

Today you're fighting mental tigers which are just as dangerous to your health and job security as the real ones. If you're going to live a long, successful, and happy life, you've got to learn how to control your tensions and aggressions. This chapter will suggest ways to help you do it.

IDEAL MENTAL FITNESS

In this context, ideal mental fitness can be defined simply as your having a positive, self-confident, and relaxed outlet on life and your work: one unimpaired by excessive frustration, aggression, and emotional stress. It sounds simple, but then not many of us live in a monastery.

HOW TO IMPROVE YOUR MENTAL FITNESS AND BUSINESS ABILITY

First, you've got to find out whether or not you're under "excessive" tensions or if you're slowly developing them. Search yourself. If you can honestly answer no to all these symptoms of tension, you're probably leading a well-adjusted and happy life. If not, you may be heading for job problems, ill health, or at least premature old age.

1. Are you over the age of thirty and frequently described as driven, overstriving, or unable to relax without pangs of guilt?

2. Do you race with the clock in everything you do?

3. Are you resentful and insecure in your work? You may be passive by nature and feel dependent on others, but do these feelings make you overcompensate with hyperactivity and aggressive behavior?

4. Do you suffer consistent mental conflict and tension and have trouble expressing feelings? Do you bottle up aggressions? Are you overcontrolled and restrained; rigidly conservative?

5. Finally, are you an "adrenaline addict"? We all have some of the adrenaline addict in us. Addicts feel best in situations of tension and exhaustive activity which forces their bodies to release adrenaline like our primitive caveman. They seem stimulated by tension in their business and private lives, enjoy aggressive confrontations, and work themselves up into fits of righteous indignation over little things. You usually find them in the more competitive and insecure professions. Advertising and sales organizations are full of them.

Where no tension normally exists, the adrenaline addict goes out of his way to create it. He leaves for work in the morning just that bit late to force himself to rush and fight traffic. He has to be the last on the airport bus so he'll be the first on the plane so he can sit by the door so he'll be the first off the plane, and so it goes right through passport control, customs, and the hotel. He calls it efficiency, but everyone else on the plane always seems to get to the hotel at the same time. His blood pressure rises from the frustration of not being able to pass another car on the road. Tension and aggression become a natural and potentially lethal part of his personality. An adrenaline addict can destroy himself—literally wear out his body bit by bit through excess tension and aggression, and insists on living in an environment that encourages him to do so.

If some or all of these traits are familiar to you, you've got a small or a big mental fitness problem. Developing a positive and relaxed approach to life and work isn't easy, but you've got to make the effort. With some thought, you can probably determine the causes of your problems, and you alone are in the best position to remove them. Treat the reduction of stress in your life as an administrative problem because that's exactly what it is. The secret is to match your daily work load and responsibilities to your mental and physical capacity. If you let them get out of balance for too long, you may crack up. These suggestions can help:

Don't identify yourself personally with every problem around you at work or at home. Don't clutter up your mind with worries that are none of your business and over which you have no control. If there's nothing you can do about a tough situation, don't fret. Adjust to it. If you can contribute to its solution, don't dither for days and postpone making the decision. When you let unsolved problems pile up, so, too, does stress.

Stop being a loner. Don't try to stand all alone as the proverbial "pillar of strength." It may be an attractive image to have for a while, but when it starts to crumble, disaster! Everyone needs someone with whom he can unbottle and discuss problems. Work with those around you and be ready to compromise, not in the quality of the work, but on how best to do it.

Delegate responsibility. This certainly doesn't come as a surprise to you. It's a cardinal rule of good management and as such should be adhered to. By delegation, you free yourself to concentrate on the more important aspects of your job while training those under you into a more productive team, which will further ease your burden and enable you to proceed up the line of command with less drain on your energy reserves.

Channel insecurities constructively. Many companies feel a bit of job insecurity stimulates their employees to perform better, but only if those insecurities are channeled properly. Men must know their efforts can succeed and that they have the support of others around them. Let the men under your supervision know how good or bad you consider their work, and help them improve it. Don't let them stew for months worrying about their future. This will land you with a weak and inefficient supporting team, and so you'll only be increasing your own work load and the drain on your time and energy.

Refuse excessive work loads. The strain of working at overcapacity for too long a time will result in mental inefficiency, counterproductive work, and serious health problems which will inevitably bring you down. Match your work load to your available energy. When taking on new responsibilities, make sure you can shed or delegate some of the old.

I'm sure you've known men who were successful and happy until promoted to positions with too much work and responsibility for their energies. After a while the tensions got so great they couldn't cope no matter how hard they tried. In fact, their performance level fell below that of their old job. Finally all that was left to them was the "golden handshake." A waste of good men.

Enjoy idleness to the fullest. Ever since we were children, society has drummed into us that work is good and idleness is bad. Working until you drop from exhaustion represented the stereotype of a "good day's work." Society, alas, was wrong. Don't drive your body and mind until you drop: stop when you get tired. Give in to fatigue and rest without feeling guilty. If you do, you'll be able to do much more work in the long run.

A business associate who used to jet from one country to another with as much ease as you'd hop in and out of taxis, trained himself to drop into a deep sleep for periods of exactly fifteen minutes. During nonproductive times like waiting for luggage, taxi trips to hotels or between meetings he'd pop off regardless of the general confusion around him. (I must admit it was a bit eerie to watch.) With a few naps under his belt during the day, he'd sail through a productive ten-hour or more work schedule with freshness and enthusiasm.

Exercise throughout the day. Tension that doesn't lead to movement can be harmful, so channel it into some form of nonstress activity during the day. As recommended in the previous chapter, stretch your muscles or do a few general fitness office exercises. Take a fast walk or do some sports at lunchtime. The sooner you exercise after periods of tension, the better. Also, the more fit you keep your body, the better it will deal with tension and the more energy you'll have for work and play.

Be calm. Do the opposite of the adrenaline addict. Administer your activities and life to create a relaxed environment. Keep some quiet place at home where you can retreat to think and read books that will broaden your interests and distract you from the problems around you. Concentrate on one thing at a time: Don't create mental conflict. Start early for appointments, linger over meals, and learn to savor good food and drink. Play cards and sports well, but not too aggressively. Save your aggression for the situations that have a more important effect on your future progress and happiness. Don't indulge in the lethal luxury of working yourself into fits of righteous indignation over things. Keep an open mind, and after you've made your point, shut up. Is it really that important that everyone agree with you on everything?

Administer well. As you will have realized, those things that contribute to your mental health and fitness at work are also the things that most management consultants recommend to increase administrative effectiveness. That's why I referred earlier to mental fitness as an administrative problem.

To simplify even more, perhaps this entire section could be summed up with the two words so popular with those who challenge many of the values of society today: "Cool it."

A WARNING AGAINST HEART ATTACKS

If you find it impossible to stop overworking and to train yourself out of tense, aggressive behavior, you may find yourself facing a potential heart attack. They seldom strike without warning, so keep your eyes open to signs that may increase in intensity over the months or years. See your doctor regularly, be honest with him about the tensions you're under, and let him keep a check on your blood pressure. Your wife will probably be the first to notice signs of stress in you, so don't snap her head off when she begs you to see the doctor.

Men have variable resistance to aggression, insecurity, and other stresses in their life. Everyone adjusts to them differently. But when you can't cope with them any longer, the following symptoms or changes in your behavior may start to appear:

- Your general health begins to deteriorate and you have an increasing tendency to contract more minor illnesses.
- You become increasingly tired; work becomes a burden and you feel the need for more rest at home each day. Getting up in the morning becomes more and more difficult.
- Physical work takes more of an effort and exercise brings heavy breathing.
- You don't sleep well, become irritable and grumbling and may develop an explosive temper.
- Your mental and business efficiency slowly degenerates. You become counterproductive, doing more work but achieving less. You have trouble dealing with and getting the cooperation of people around you.

- You may feel frustrated and persecuted, talk and gripe more than usual about company problems.
- You tend to smoke, drink, and eat too much.

Faced with this rather unattractive list, don't you think it's worth a little effort to get your tensions and aggressions under control? I'm sure those around you do.

Chapter 19

Sleep: The Rejuvenating Effects of This Twilight World

You've seen how important your physical and mental fitness can be to an active, happy, and successful life, but what role does sleep play? What happens during that third of every day you spend in darkness and dreams?

Sleep isn't the simple thing you may think. Your brain doesn't lie unconscious while your head lies on the pillow; quite the opposite. It keeps control over your body, altering its functions to adjust to dream phantoms that glide through your shadow world and monitoring the real world outside to rouse you into action when necessary. Each night, you drift back and forth between two types of sleep, one associated with the repair and maintenance of your body cells, the other more with your brain cells. You need the right amount of each.

Too little or too much sleep affects your mental efficiency and rationality, your health, and your outlook on life. There's nothing to be proud about in sleeping fewer hours than your friends and in driving yourself to do so. Scientists have scratched only the surface of the chemistry and behavior of your brain in relation to its patterns of sleep. Nevertheless, what they've learned from this scratch tells us not to underestimate the role of sleep in a long and successful life.

MAKING SURE YOU GET THE PROPER AMOUNT OF SLEEP

You need only enough sleep to satisfy the needs of your own individual body and brain, no more. Under normal, unrestricted conditions your body will find its natural rhythm of sleep and activity. Respect that rhythm.

Set aside enough time for sleep every day

Every night you need relatively fixed proportions of two types of sleep: orthodox sleep and paradoxical (REM) sleep. If you don't get enough of one today, you make up by taking more of it tomorrow. This has been attributed to your brain's need to retain some unknown, internal chemical balance.

Orthodox sleep has been linked to the time especially important to the restoration of many of the tissues of your body. During deep orthodox sleep, the amount of growth hormone in your blood increases. It may be no coincidence that the rate of cell division in some tissues (skin and bone marrow) increases just before or during sleep when the increased levels of growth hormone are present to aid new cell growth.

Sleep-deprived men and those of you who, by nature, sleep fewer hours than average take more orthodox sleep. It appears that the more energy you use up during the day, the more of this deep sleep you need at night. The intensity of orthodox sleep is deeper in the first two hours of sleep than the last two, so it probably has greater restorative power in the few hours just after you retire.

Paradoxical sleep appears linked to dreams and the restoration and development of your brain. You usually spend one and a half to two hours in this type of sleep every night.

Inappropriate or damaged brain cells must constantly be replaced or renewed. During paradoxical sleep, more blood flows through your brain than during waking hours and the brain's heat output rises. Both represent signs of increased chemical activity in your brain cells similar to that needed for protein synthesis and cell growth. Adult senility (the symptoms of which may start in your early thirties) is accompanied by a decline in paradoxical sleep. In senile decay the processes of cell renewal decline and the brain actually shrivels.

To determine how much sleep you need and establish the proper sleeping pattern, start by setting aside eight hours from the time you turn off the light until the alarm goes off in the morning. Stay in bed the full eight hours. If your body and brain don't need all that sleep, after a few weeks or so you can start cutting down the time. Let your body, not your social schedule, set the pattern. It's all right if a few late parties break the pattern as long as you pick up the lost sleep the next night. Use your common sense and don't bend the rules too far. After all, it's your brain that has to be clear the next day, and it's your health.

Under conditions of extreme sleep deprivation for a period of several days, you can lose your ability for sustained concentration. Your thinking has a dreamlike quality, becomes irrational, and you find yourself unable to effectively relate past experiences to the solution of current new problems. The brainwashing technique uses extreme sleep deprivation to so isolate the victim from his lifetime of experiences and accepted principles that he can be swayed to embrace new and seemingly logical concepts that would previously have been alien to him.

Men who make a habit of not getting enough sleep lower their resistance to infectious illness and become irritable. They impair their business efficiency as well as their ability to enjoy life.

Don't take tension to bed with you

While you sleep, your brain continues to direct your body's internal functions just as when awake, and presumably dream stimuli affect brain action just as real life stimuli do. It has been found that the more anxiety in a dream, the greater the level of adrenaline-released free fatty acids in the dreamer's bloodstream. Ulcer sufferers have experienced increases in stomach acids during high-activity dreams.

There's some indication that stress and tension experienced prior to sleeping may help put your brain in a state of turmoil and anxiety which manifests itself in more active, vivid, and emotional dreams. Thus, stress can put a strain on your cardiovascular and other support systems not only during the day but while you sleep. Corny as it may sound, think calm, happy thoughts before settling down for the night.

Spend half an hour or so relaxing, doing things involving rhythmic stimulation like listening to soothing music, reading a not too fascinating book in bed or in a rocking chair. If worries still press in on you, try to blot them out. Some men use the television, others force themselves to think of pleasant things. They plan vacations, pretend they've all the money in the world and spend it on remodeling their homes, buying yachts, or flying off to Shangri-La. This could be a good time for you to memorize some foreign language vocabulary. A friend used to read a page from the almanac every night before sleep and may truly be said to possess one of the world's most boring gold mines of meaningless information.

So you think you don't dream? It's generally accepted that the normal man dreams as much as one and a half to two hours every night, usually during periods of paradoxical sleep. A dream is a fantasy life in which you actively participate. It doesn't happen in a flash, as was once thought, but extends through time. Most men think of dreams only as wild, fanciful things, and don't count or forget the ones that can be quite ordinary, like real-life situations and events which happen day after day. That's why, if you can't recall something extraordinary, you probably think you haven't dreamed at all. Also, unless roused during or just at the end of a dream, you'll seldom remember anything about it.

A great deal has been written and hypothesized on this subject, and naturally disagreement exists on various aspects of dream analysis, and the functions, benefits, and dangers to the mind of dreams and dream deprivation. Some experts claim that depriving people of dreams would reduce them to a state of neurosis in which they couldn't function effectively. Some say we get rid of or sublimate anxieties and problems by exposing and dealing with them in this fantasy world. Rather than go into a detailed and lengthy discussion of things over which you have little or no practical control, I believe it sufficient to say that the psychological value of dreams to your mental health is obviously very great, so dream on. . . .

What happens when you're not dreaming? A lot of evidence points to the fact that when you're not dreaming, mental life of another sort goes on throughout the night. During periods of orthodox sleep, your brain can probably be said to be in a "thinking" state, mulling over the mundane events of the previous day.

When roused from sleep during these times, men usually say they haven't been dreaming or thinking about anything. They attribute what may be lingering in their minds to the remembrance of something they were thinking about before falling asleep. Yet while in this "thinking" state, the intensity of electrical impulses on their skin surface has been found to fluctuate depending upon the severity of the anxiety they experienced during the preceding day. Another reminder of the effects emotional stress can have on your mind and body.

Try to avoid taking sleeping pills

Use sleeping pills only as a temporary aid to restoring your natural sleeping pattern. Let your doctor help you with this. Many people (women more than men) become physically and psychologically addicted to sleeping pills and need increasing amounts as their body's tolerance to these drugs increases. (See Chapter 22.)

Some men naturally sleep better than others. They sleep more and wake less often during the night. They fall asleep sooner, their body temperatures fall lower, and their hearts beat more slowly. These men tend to take more paradoxical sleep and are less prone to worries and personality problems which inhibit sleep. This may be one reason why extroverts sleep better than introverts, who are more emotionally bottled up. Pills won't solve this basic problem.

Young men sleep better than older ones. Starting at the age of about thirty, sleep begins to deteriorate. It's normal for older people to sleep less and wake more often at night. A gradual change shouldn't cause alarm.

You're sleeping better than you think. You always hear complaints from friends about sleepless nights, yet they've probably slept most of the night without realizing it. While asleep you lose track of time. Therefore, a few scattered periods of agonizing wakefulness when you toss and hear the hall clocks chiming seem much longer and more vivid than those blank hours of sleep you've actually enjoyed. If an older person appears spry throughout the day, chances are he slept pretty well the night before, no matter what he says to the contrary.

Get up when you wake up

If you've had your normal amount of sleep, get up when you wake. Too much sleep can be almost as bad for you as too little. Sleeping a few extra hours a day may have detrimental effects on your efficiency and alertness and produce a feeling of grogginess. If you often feel drowsy all day, think twice about whether you're getting too little or too much sleep.

Psychologically, some men stay in bed longer and find it harder to get up because they basically don't want to face another anxious day. I'm sure you've had those mornings when you leaped from bed refreshed and ready to plunge into some pleasant activity, in contrast to those when you clung desperately to a few extra minutes of sleep trying to postpone the problems of the approaching day. By creating a relaxed and happy work environment, you'll find it a lot easier to get up in the mornings. It takes us right back to mental fitness and administering your life to get the most out of it.

Think positive and optimistic thoughts

Thinking positively as soon as you open your eyes will set a happier and more constructive tone to your entire day. Not only will your office productivity be greatly improved, but those around you will be more appreciative and co-operative. No one likes to work with a "loser."

Of course, some men have trouble doing this. A classmate once asked our psychology professor how he could brighten his normally pessimistic outlook on life. The professor advised him to sing the happiest song he knew every morning upon rising. The following week, when asked how this approach was working, the student replied despondently that hard as he'd tried, he just couldn't think of a happy song so early in the morning.

AN ADDED BONUS: BE A BETTER SPEAKER

Understanding the science of sleep, various levels of mental consciousness, and the effects of monotony can help you speak much better before an audience.

Your level of consciousness at any given time is that level of efficiency with which your brain can carry out creative activity. The lowest level of consciousness or vigilance occurs while asleep. Your brain is pepped up just enough to keep a minimal scrutiny on its exterior environment. Significant changes in that environment—a baby's cry, the creaking of a floorboard—feed into your brain's computers which decide what action to take: whether to sleep on, or to leap from bed ready to defend life and limb.

Going up the vigilance scale, you pass through the state of drowsiness where your mind is fuzzy, filled with vague dreamlike images and disconnected thoughts. It can't support an effort of concentration. On this level your mind can't learn or grasp anything new. How many times have you nodded over the same paragraph in your evening paper without comprehending a single word until you roused yourself into greater alertness? You've got to keep your audience from slipping into this fuzzy state.

From drowsiness you rise up through ever increasing levels of consciousness until you reach the optimum level, the point at which your brain can calmly and efficiently deal with all the stimuli and problems at hand. This is where you want to keep your audience. The optimum level varies. The more work and sensory stimuli the brain has to handle, the higher its corresponding level of vigilance—up to a point.

The highest level is too high. Your brain can't work efficiently and becomes confused because it's overstimulated with too many impulses and its attention is directed in too many areas. It can't absorb things or concentrate on any one thing long enough to deal with it effectively. Remember those confused times when you were late leaving for the airport, the taxi hadn't arrived, your report was still being typed, and you couldn't find your tickets or passport. What kind of coherent answers was your brain able to come up with for those men who popped in with last-minute questions? Probably something like, "Can't it wait?" or "How the hell should I know?" Bearing this in mind, don't make your audience's brains work so hard trying to follow you that they lose track and click off. Take them from point to point gradually and rationally. Don't skip about.

Monotony reduces your level of vigilance. Men inherit varying tendencies to drowse, but even the most alert have trouble fighting against monotony which, in conjunction with restricted movement, acts to slowly lower their level of vigilance to that of drowsiness or sleep. Surprisingly, monotonous things of potential interest induce sleep more effectively than conditions of meaningless uniformity. Watching a repeated pattern of blinking lights usually brings sleep faster than sitting quietly in a dark room. This most certainly creates problems for the speaker trying to capture and educate his audience.

Remember that you're starting out with several strikes against you. First, your audience has potential interest in your subject; second, their movements are pretty much restricted for a considerable period of time; and finally, you have only one voice, one accent, and one tone. As a result, no matter how good a speaker you consider yourself, you're almost sure to put some people to sleep and many others into a level of uncomprehending drowsiness.

Stage-manage your speech to break its inherent monotony and keep the vigilance level of your audience high by constantly sending it unique and new stimuli.

- Aside from your spoken voice, stimulate the eyes and ears of your audience with slides, films, charts, sound effects, and the like.
- Vary the lighting in the room and, if possible, never speak in the dark with only yourself and the screen illuminated for more than a few minutes.
- When using visual aids, change the length of time each is shown so you don't establish a monotonous rhythm like one slide following smoothly on top of the other, over and over

again. Try two slow slides, then three fast ones, etc., to keep the pace broken and the audience mind alert.

- If possible, vary the moods of your talk, part serious and part light, happy and sad, pretty and ugly.
- Try for some audience participation. Throw out easy questions or invite comment and questions from the floor. Break up long speaking sessions with some periods for active stretching, coffee, and the like.

These represent just some of the monotony-breaking tools you can bring to bear on your audience to get the attention they most sincerely want to give you. But in breaking the monotony, make sure you don't overstimulate and confuse their brains. All these tools should fit naturally into the progression of your speech as it moves logically from one point to the next and on to your conclusion.

Try a little voodoo at your local discothèque

Investigating the various levels of your mental consciousness can be interesting. Dance rhythms accompanied by hand clapping, foot stamping, or repeated visual stimuli can lower your vigilance level so far that you fall into a half sleep or trance. In this state you're prone to see dreamlike images, hear voices, all the things we associate with voodoo ritual. Next time you're at your favorite discothèque, don't talk with your partner—make a blank of your mind and concentrate on the music. After dancing for some time to the loud, pounding beat and flashing strobe lights, see if you don't experience the unreal floating feeling found in a state of trance. It can be a unique sensation.

CHAPTER 20

Feet: How to Keep Yours Healthy and Strong

You probably neglect your feet more than any part of your body. As long as they don't call attention to themselves by itching, smelling, or pain, you think they're healthy and happy. This can be a very short-term view. Long term, you may be damning yourself to a pair of weak, aching feet, unable to support and carry you about as well as you might want. The general who said an army marches on its belly lost the war.

Keeping your feet healthy and better-looking doesn't take any time at all; you just have to know what you're doing.

THE IDEAL FOOT

Apparently the perfect pair of men's feet exists only on the idealized statues of ancient Greece, but even these feet don't fit today's criteria. The Greeks considered a foot truly beautiful only if the second toe were longer than the first. On the average twentieth-century foot, the big toe is the longest and the other four progressively shorter. (To prove the point of neglect, I'll bet you can't remember which of your toes is longest.) Fortunately, there's agreement on six criteria for healthy, good-looking feet.

They should carry you about or support you in a standing position during the day without undue fatigue or aching. Their bone structure must be flexible (not stiff or arthritic) and the ligaments and muscles, strong and pliable.

Your arches should be well defined when you stand (although flat feet aren't the villains we once thought).

Toes are normally shaped, flexible, point straight forward, and don't curl inward when you walk.

The skin feels supple, smooth, and naturally dry (neither damp and clammy nor overly dry and flaky). There should be no areas of hardened skin like calluses or corns, and no irritation or fungal diseases.

Your toenails, like fingernails, should grow freely over their nail beds and within the grooves of flesh at the sides to the tip of each toe where they're cut relatively flat across. They are smooth, strong, and flexible, pink and free of discoloration. The cuticles are smooth and even and can be lifted slightly from the nails.

Last but not least, your feet should have a **clean, natural footy smell,** not the offensive odor associated with sweat and bacterial action.

THE PROPER WAY TO CARE FOR YOUR FEET

Lots of us could have danced all night or walked a mile for that fabled cigarette, but not with aching feet. You're not relaxed and at your best anywhere if your feet hurt, smell, or you're busy trying to cover them up with sand at the beach. Use this simple regimen to keep them strong and healthy, and to make them more attractive. It shouldn't take any time at all, just a little thought.

1. Stop falling arches

The treatment for falling arches is twofold: first, get rid of the pain and discomfort they cause, and second, stop them from falling farther by strengthening your foot and leg muscles.

Your feet have three and a half arches to give them the flexibility and strength needed to support and move your weight. Two run the length of your foot from the first three toes to your heel (the inner longitudinal arch) and from the last two toes to the heel (the outer longitudinal arch). The third is an arch across the joints of your toes (the anterior metatarsal arch), and the half arch (the transverse arch) runs over the center of your foot. When you put both feet together, your arches form a domelike space beneath.

A **flat foot** is one with a weak or fallen arch. It's a very common ailment which need not cause you much difficulty if dealt with correctly. You can see for yourself whether or not you've got flat feet by looking at your footprints. The normal, preferred foot has a well-defined arch, and so its print looks narrower in the middle (a). As your arches weaken, the center width of the print widens (b) until, with flat feet, it's almost the same from heel to toe (c).

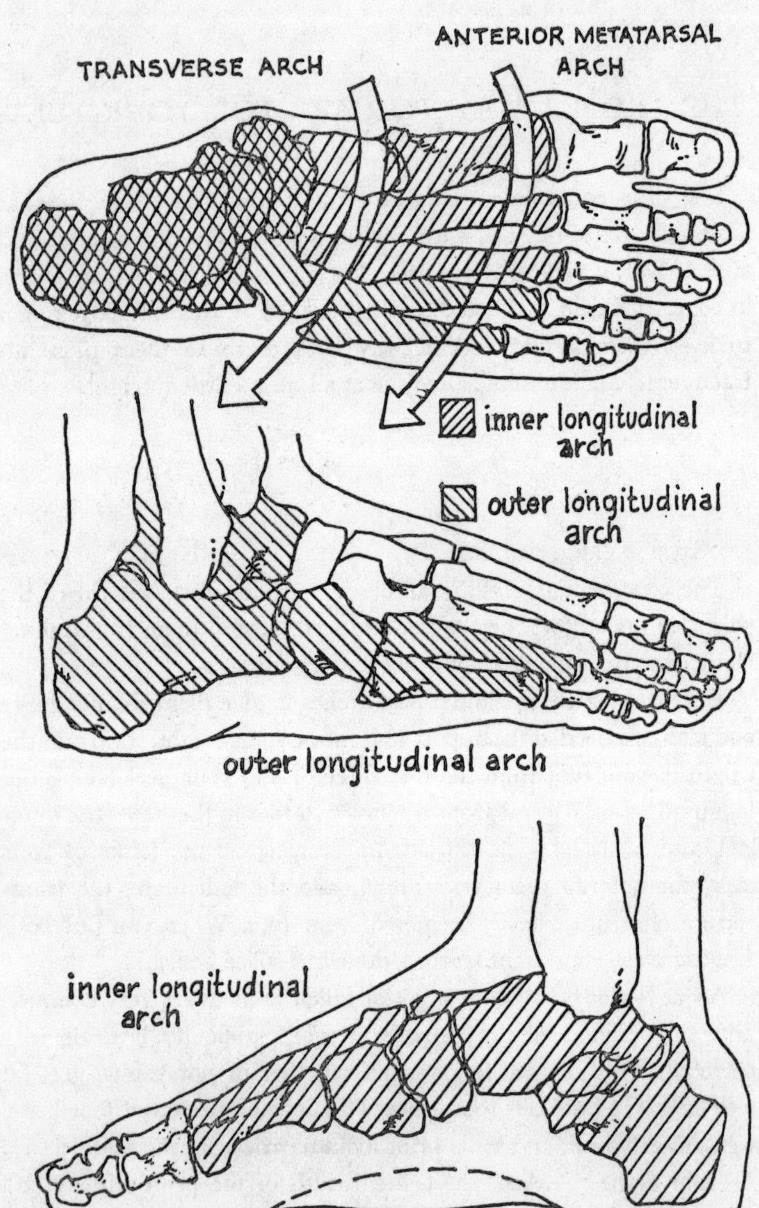
ANTERIOR METATARSAL ARCH
TRANSVERSE ARCH
inner longitudinal arch
outer longitudinal arch
outer longitudinal arch
inner longitudinal arch

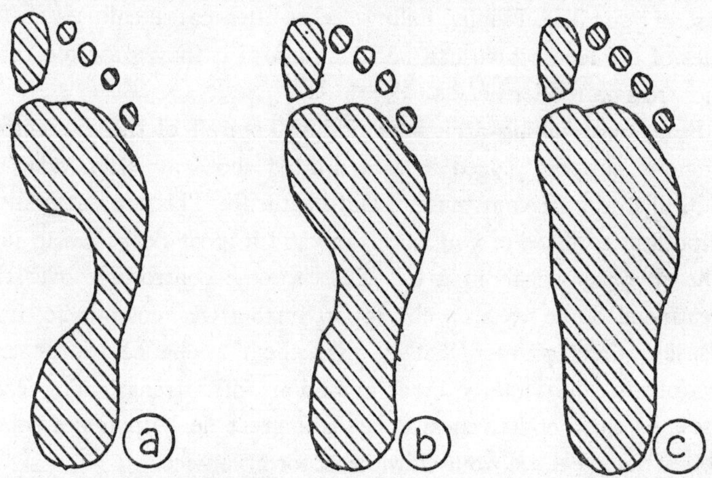

The cause of flat feet can be injury, rheumatic conditions like arthritis, and bad shoes. Poor posture and over-all weak leg and feet muscles which fail to hold up the arches take much of the blame, as do overweight, carrying heavy loads, or standing still for long periods of time, all of which strain good muscles and ligaments. Unlike muscles, ligaments don't have great flexibility, and if stretched too far, can't return to their original shorter length and so give less and less support to your arches.

Flat feet are not necessarily bad. African natives living on the plains usually have feet flat as pancakes yet run like gazelles without apparent discomfort.

The problem appears to lie not with *fallen* arches, but with *falling* arches which cause fatigue and aching in your legs and feet because the supporting muscles and ligaments (which run through the foot on up through the lower leg) are being stretched and strained every time you stand or walk. As they're not strong enough to support and hold the arches in place, your foot bones can jar together to create pain over and under your arches. You may also experience a dull, dragging pain in your heel caused by the overstretching of the tissue connecting the base of your heel with the base of your toes. Finally, falling arches often cause calluses on the soles of the feet, which can become painful if they grow too thick and press on tender nerves.

First, treat falling arches by ridding yourself of the discomfort. An arch support placed in a well-fitted shoe can often take the painful strain off your muscles and ligaments. This support is more important to those of you who stand still a great deal than to men who sit or move about a lot. There's some controversy over this treatment. Some say an arch support further weakens muscles from disuse; others counter that it gives them a chance to rest and recuperate, particularly in combination with strengthening exercises. As their effectiveness depends a great deal upon the condition of your feet, ask your chiropodist for his advice.

You can relieve tired and aching feet and leg muscles by increasing blood circulation to carry off the waste by-products of their activity. Walking and simple foot exercises will increase circulation, but massage appears most effective; certainly more effective than soaking your feet in warm water.

Second, strengthen foot and leg muscles with proper exercise to keep your arches from falling farther. If caught in time, some experts believe it's possible to actually correct or improve an arch by strengthening the muscles before the ligaments are stretched out of shape.

Keep your leg muscles strong with some of the exercises in Appendix 4. In most cases, walking properly, particularly barefoot on firm surfaces, will strengthen both leg and foot muscles. When you walk, your body weight should be distributed throughout your feet to increase their efficiency of movement and minimize fatigue. Your heel touches ground first and bears the initial weight. As your body moves directly over the foot, support of its weight moves along the outside of the outer longitudinal arch to the base of the little toe, and then across the ball of your foot. At the moment of takeoff when your body continues forward, the big toe takes the weight followed across the metatarsal arch by your other four toes. They press flat down, forcing up your arch and taking your weight off the ball of the foot.

The wrong position and movement of your toes while walking can create problems. If, because of bad habits or shoe construction, your toes curl inward while walking, too much weight falls on the ball of your foot, creating calluses and sometimes nerve pain (metatarsalgia) there.

The old trick of picking up pencils or wads of paper with your toes will exercise your arches to some extent, but also encourages your toes to curl under, which you want to avoid.

Exercise sandals have become very popular because they exercise your feet without conscious effort on your part. Their form supports your arch while you stand and forces you to walk properly by preventing your toes from curling inward. Because they're made of wood or other heavy materials, their weight provides needed resistance against toe movement to strengthen your arch and toe muscles.

Other types of sandals with toe thongs or flopping slippers usually need some toe movement to keep them from falling off, but the lightness of their construction may not give enough resistance and their flat soles can encourage shuffling and other bad walking habits. Because most of them offer little or no arch support, you might as well go barefoot.

2. Always wear good-fitting shoes

Take enough time and care in selecting your shoes. Don't consider it feminine to try on lots of different pairs and bitch about their fit. Bad-fitting shoes cause misshapen toes, structural foot problems, corns, calluses, aches and pains. With the price of shoes today, you don't have to do the salesman a favor by taking the first pair he shows you with that worn-out promise "They'll feel fine as soon as you break them in" or the excuse "With your feet, you'll never find a better fit." Thirty minutes spent on choosing the right shoe can mean years of comfort.

A proper-fitting shoe gives you gentle support *and* allows natural foot movement. Look for four things:

- Firm, but gentle, support of your arch when you stand up; you may not necessarily feel it while sitting.
- A firm fit all around the heel (not just at the top) to eliminate slipping and friction.
- There should be no restrictive pressure on your toes so they're free to move up and down, extend forward, and fan out a bit at the sides.
- The shoe should bend at the same place your foot bends. Most constructions force a shoe to bend at the broadest point along its sole. The bend of one shoe brand or style may not coincide with the bend along the ball of your foot, but certainly others will. Look until you find the right match. Of course in time your feet will force almost any shoe to fit their bends and contours, but why go through all that agony and take the chance of harming yourself?

What do you look for in shoe construction? Aside from style, your shoes should be durable, have no inner surfaces that cause friction or put undue pressure on your feet, and breathe to encourage air circulation.

Today properly cured leather is generally considered the best material for the upper part of your shoes. Being animal skin, it breathes well through its pores and is flexible and durable. Until recently manufacturers thought it best for shoe soles as well, but unfortunately it swells when wet, can let water in (usually where it joins the upper), may crack, and doesn't wear all that well. As it's not so important for the soles of shoes to breathe, some better materials are often used for soles. These resin-based materials can be bonded firmly to leather uppers, won't let water in, swell, or crack, and they have greater durability. However, they should be combined with a porous and moisture-absorbing innersole which won't support bacteria growth.

Make sure your shoes are lined in all areas where the leather or stitching threatens to cause skin abrasion. By running your fingers over the interior, you should be able to detect potential trouble areas.

Plastic or synthetic material shoes can be tricky. Some plastics breathe, but not as well as leather. Some of the cheaper ones may be completely nonporous. If you're buying trendy boots and shoes, be sure they're not made from these natural-looking but inferior materials which inhibit circulation and trap sweat and odor. Because of their construction, high boots must limit air circulation, so at least make sure yours are made of leather.

Take proper care of your shoes by airing them at night. Use shoe trees which don't interfere with air circulation and lay your shoes on their sides to help the soles dry and increase ventilation within. If your feet perspire a great deal, wear a different pair on alternate days and spray the interiors from time to time with a germicidal product to keep them from smelling. Obviously, protect your shoes from wet weather conditions and keep them polished to prolong their useful life.

3. Keep your feet feeling fresh and odor free

Wash your feet at least once a day with soap and warm, not hot, water and rinse in cold water.

Douse them with alcohol (diluted with water if your skin is inflamed) or an alcohol lotion or spray as a preventative if you've been exposed to athlete's foot or other fungal diseases at public swimming pools, showers, or clubs. You may want to make this a daily part of your foot-care regimen because of its pleasant tonic effect.

Dust your feet with a foot powder containing a bacteriostat to get rid of moisture, give more friction-free movement between your toes, and inhibit bacterial action. *Don't* use a body talcum powder on your feet because its particles may be too small and clog your pores.

If you have a foot odor problem, use a foot deodorant or antiperspirant and undertake the treatment recommended in the next chapter.

Change your socks daily and wear ones made of 100 per cent cotton or wool which help air circulate and absorb moisture. Wool socks reinforced in the heels and toes with strong synthetic fiber are a practical second choice.

If you have a foot disease or a serious foot odor problem (bromidrosis), disinfect your socks before wearing them. Wool should be washed in a disinfectant and cotton can be boiled without damaging the fabric.

4. Pedicure

Pedicure your nails and feet whenever needed to keep them looking attractive, particularly if you spend a lot of time on the beach. Surprisingly, your toenails are usually more sensitive than your fingernails, so go easy.

a. Clip your nails level with the tips of your toes and straight across (slightly rounded if you're careful). This is done more for your protection than for cosmetic reasons. Some toenails curve under at the sides. If you were to cut them in an arc, you might create two hidden nail spikes, one on each side, which could dig into the soft flesh, causing pain and possible infection. These spikes would be visible if you could flatten out the nail.

b. File your nail edges smooth with an emery board in downward strokes, making sure you don't abrade your skin. Round any sharp edges a bit so they won't bite into other toes. Leave the sides of the nails alone to encourage the flesh of the nail grooves to enfold them.

c. As you would for the cuticles of your fingernails, gently lift the toenail cuticles with a hoofstick and trim them only if necessary. Gently scrape away any acid deposits on the nail.

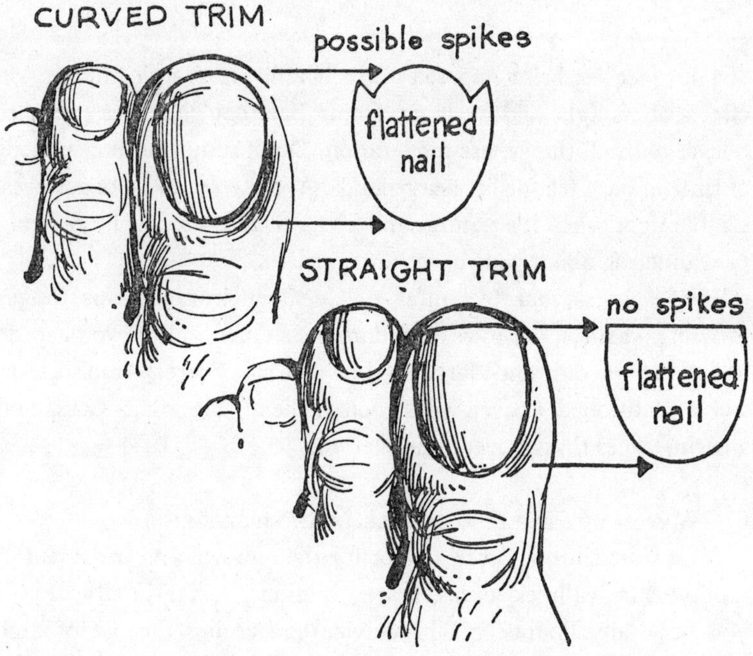

This is best done after bathing when your skin is soft and more supple.

d. Clean the free edges of your nails with cream or alcohol-saturated cotton wrapped around an orange stick. Be careful not to detach your nails from their beds. Don't use a nail file except with great caution.

e. Rub your feet with alcohol or friction lotion. File down any hard skin, calluses, and corns with the coarse side of an emery board or skin rasp. Do this gradually over a period of time to make sure you don't injure your skin. Try to remove the friction and pressure that causes these conditions.

f. If your skin appears dry and flaky or has hardened patches, rub in a foot cream. Remove any excess cream before using foot powder or putting on your shoes and socks. (Don't use a cream if you have an athlete's foot problem.)

5. Let your feet breathe

Your feet like being exposed to the healthy, antiseptic, and drying effects of sunlight and fresh air. Going barefoot gives this exposure but, as with all things, use moderation. Don't stand for long periods of time in bare feet or lift heavy loads. Avoid cold and wet surfaces. Go barefoot when it's natural and pleasant to do so, while relaxing or wandering about your house and garden.

Inside shoes, your feet offer the ideal environment for fungus growth: warmth, darkness, and dampness. There's little you can do about the warmth and darkness, but you can decrease moisture as we've mentioned above, with good hygiene, the right socks, and wearing shoes that allow air circulation.

6. Watch out for foot problems and disease

Visit your chiropodist or doctor for the removal and treatment of troublesome calluses, corns, warts, bunions, and skin diseases. If you have any doubts, get his advice concerning the use of arch supports and exercise sandals and going barefoot. You may have an unusual foot condition which requires special treatment.

FOOT PROBLEMS, DISEASES, AND TREATMENT

Calluses

This hardening of your skin results from friction and pressure. Sometime calluses become premanent, and no matter how often they're removed, the hard epidermis grows back.

Aside from not being particularly attractive, calluses don't cause much trouble unless they become extreme and press painfully against nerve endings.

You treat calluses by removing the friction and pressure that causes them, and then removing the calluses themselves. If relatively minor, you can abrade them away with an emery board or skin rasp. More serious ones should be handled by a chiropodist.

Corns

Corns are basically smaller and more intense calluses caused by greater friction and pressure on a smaller area. Corns are a hardening of your epidermis with a clearly defined conical nucleus which points inward from your skin surface. Pain results when the nucleus presses on your nerve endings.

Like calluses, attack both the cause and the effect. The cause can often be removed by a shoe change, the corn by your chiropodist. Protective corn pads may ease pain temporarily, but they're just transferring the offending pressure to a larger area.

Bunions

A series of steps, each of which may or may not be painful, go into making a bunion. Poor-fitting shoes can force your big toe into a position where pressure falls on the joint of its base. This causes a bone growth to develop and then a burse (a sac of jellylike fluid) to form between the growth and skin surface. When this entire construction becomes inflamed, you've got a first-class bunion. Inflammation, however, may accompany any of the preceding steps.

Again, your chiropodist is best equipped to remove the bunion; you the cause.

Verruca

This viral wart is caused by the inoculation of the virus into your skin through a small tear or by scratching. It grows into the surface of the epidermis which becomes horny and may be very painful under pressure, particularly on the soles of your feet or when touched by your shoe.

Sometimes pain can be relieved by using a hollow ring of felt to protect the wart until it disappears, but you may need surgery to remove it more quickly.

Bony spur

Bony spur often results from falling arches. It's a bone growth which develops in the shape of a shelf extending from the base of your heel toward the toes, parallel with the ground. As your arches fall, the heel leans forward and the spur tilts to the ground, exposing itself to painful pressure.

By elevating your arch with a support, you can often tilt the spur back up and so reduce or eliminate the pain. Heel cushions are sometimes used in the shoe. In extreme cases, you may have to resort to surgery to remove the spur.

Ingrown toenails

Ingrown toenails result from nails that you've trimmed improperly or from incorrectly shaped and fitted shoes.

The usual treatment is to wedge thin rolls of lamb's wool soaked in natural oil (olive oil or lanolin) between the side grooves of flesh and your nail until it grows out to its proper shape.

Athlete's foot

"Athlete's foot" is the popular name for a fungal infection (*Tinea pedis*) which can develop between your toes and on your soles and spreads back over the feet if not contained. The fungus thrives on warm, moist skin and in the dark conditions inside your shoes. It's highly contagious, often picked up from damp floors in public pool and gymnasiums, and can be spread to other parts of your body by scratching.

The infected skin is white, macerated, and often split, like a paper tissue soaked in water and pulled slowly apart. Or it may be red and inflamed. Your skin feels itchy and sometimes sore.

The treatment involves killing the fungus and its spores and drying the infected area. A liquid formulation containing a borotannic complex in an alcohol base has proved very effective in curing athlete's foot. When painted on the infected area every twelve hours, it kills the surface fungus, makes the pH level of your skin more acid to discourage fungal growth, and penetrates deep into the tissues to kill the spores. The formula also has a drying action to stop maceration, and it reduces irritation.

The use of foot powder and exposing your feet to sunlight and air during treatment help keep the skin dry. Obviously your socks should be changed daily and disinfected.

Cream medicaments don't appear to be as effective as the liquid paints in treating this condition because the creams may trap some moisture in the skin, and they take time to penetrate deep enough to kill the spores. You should refer any serious or lingering case to your doctor.

Perspiration in extreme forms can also cause maceration of the skin and should not be confused, as it so often is, with athlete's foot or other similar conditions. To cure this problem, keep your feet dry and use powders and medicaments that have a drying effect.

Ringworm

Ringworm has nothing to do with worms; it's another fungal infection in the tinea group. On relatively hairless skin, the infection takes the form of a slowly expanding ring of inflammation, looking red and scaly, with an active edge which may contain tiny blisters. This infection can often be found in one's groin and on the thighs.

The treatment is similar to that for athlete's foot: killing the fungus and its spores and keeping your skin dry. Various ointments and liquid paints exist to counter the infection, and your pharmacist should be able to suggest one. If the inflammation persists after you've treated it, see your doctor.

Onychomycosis

This fungal infection causes deterioration and a white, yellow, or yellow-brown discoloration on part or all of your nail. It's rarely painful and can often be treated with stronger versions of the athlete's foot medicaments. Cure may take from three to eighteen months.

Onychomycosis looks very unattractive and can be difficult to cure once it gets a good foothold. A friend has such a bad case that his wife won't let him on the beach without his tennis shoes. She's not all that happy about getting into bed with it either.

CHAPTER 21

Body Odor from Head to Toe: How to Stop It

Every living thing on earth gives out its own unique smell, but somewhere along the line, we *Homo sapiens* decided not to. Hamsters rub their bodies over objects to leave their scent of ownership. The smell of a female in heat arouses the male of her species to amazing feats. The greatest sex sham must be that which is perpetrated by some flowers who lure bees to cross-pollinate them by duplicating the bee's "ready and willing" sex scent. The contrary occurs with us.

Business, social, and sexual success in our sophisticated society demands the absence of any form of body odor except those we buy in bottles and jars. Ironically, we're just substituting our own sex smells for those of the civet, musk deer, and beaver, whose glands form the fixative agents in fragrances and perfumes.

Since success means getting rid of odor, then get rid of it we must. But where to begin? About 95 per cent of your body odor comes from relatively small areas: your hair, underarms, crotch, and feet. Let's start at the top.

HAIR ODOR

THE CAUSES

When clean, your hair and scalp have a delicate natural smell, normally quite pleasing. But your 100,000 or more strands of hair covered with scalp oil behave like a filter to trap dust and every smell carried in the air, particularly cigarette smoke and cooking odors.

THE TREATMENT

The answer to this problem is simple. Just shampoo your hair regularly. Consult Chapter 2.

Massaging your scalp with mildly scented friction lotion (basically alcohol, water, and perfume) will give your hair a pleasant, light smell that may mask odors for a day or two. Also check the strength and type of fragrance in your shampoo, hair lotion, or cream to make sure it's one your woman will find appealing; not too overpowering.

MOUTH ODOR—HALITOSIS

THE CAUSES

Bad breath may be caused by conditions in your mouth, stomach, or both. Foul breath can come from decaying teeth and bad gums (pyorrhea) as well as poor oral hygiene, inadequate brushing, and failure to clean away plaque and decaying food debris. Eating garlic and similar odorific foods represents only a temporary and easily avoidable cause of bad breath.

Radical dietary changes, constipation, and other stomach upsets can land you with major halitosis problems. Your nervous system also gives a helping hand by drying out your mouth and throat in times of tension, so your breath turns sour.

Treating mouth odor

Because of its many causes, the means of fighting bad breath are varied. The base treatment relies on maintaining good health with proper diet, exercise, and relaxation. Add regular visits to your dentist to eliminate odor from tooth decay and gum disease. Daily attention to oral hygiene (see Chapter 7) can reduce halitosis by keeping your teeth and mouth as clean and fresh as possible. If you can't brush after eating, at least rinse your mouth thoroughly.

Do mouthwashes stop bad breath? They have a transient deodorant effect on the oral causes of bad breath, but little or no effect on the others. Well-formulated mouthwashes are designed to temporarily freshen your mouth, reduce odor from bad teeth and gums, and kill or inhibit the action of destructive oral bacteria. They're primarily oral antiseptics. Liquid brands usually contain a mixture of flavors and odorants like menthol and eucalyptole in a base of glycerin, alcohol, and water.

Mouthwashes walk a delicate line between killing germs and overkilling them. It may take years of formulation and testing before one can be judged effective for public use. The many different bacteria living in your mouth constantly war to keep each other in check. Should an oral antiseptic kill too many of the "good" bacteria while attacking the "bad," all hell can break loose.

Well-formulated and tested mouthwashes, when used according to instructions, should give no cause for concern and can help you fight bad breath. The duration of their deodorant effect depends to a great extent on the strength and type of their antibacterial formulation, the odor-masking ability of their flavors, and the amount of saliva and food passing through your mouth. In passing, don't be fooled into thinking that a strong-tasting mouthwash is necessarily more effective than a pleasant-tasting one. Taste doesn't kill germs.

Other aids for sweeter breath

For instant help, try one of the various products in spray or tablet form that sweeten or freshen your breath more by masking mouth odor with strong flavors than by inhibiting oral bacteria. They're good for what they are, but attack the effect rather than the cause.

Gum and similar chewing or sucking products help fight bad breath by stimulating the flow of saliva and thereby keep your mouth moist and, to some extent, freer of decaying food particles. Just make sure these products don't contain much sugar or you'll be swapping bad breath for tooth decay.

BODY ODOR—B.O.

The causes

You have more bacteria living on the surface of your skin than there are people on this earth. Body odor comes primarily from these bacteria which thrive and multiply on the materials contained in your perspiration.

You exude two types of perspiration from about 2.5 million pores scattered over your body:

- Under your arms and in the pubic area, the sweat contains protein and fatty material which odor-causing bacteria love.
- In nonpubic areas your sweat is virtually pure salt water and so offers little comfort to skin bacteria. Hence little odor exists on the rest of your body surface with the exception of your feet, which have a different problem.

Aside from bacterial causes, rancid odor is caused by the oxidation of the fat in sweat when it comes into contact with the air. This represents only a minor part of body odor for most of us, but some unfortunate men literally sweat fat (not only in greater than normal quantities but in type), against which deodorants are helpless. Oxidation takes place unchecked, and they suffer very strong and repellent body odor.

Sweating and its consequent odor can often be made worse by overweight, eating highly spiced foods, and drinking stimulants like coffee and alcohol. I often see a brilliant, plump expatriate writer in many of London's curry restaurants with glass raised in one hand and dripping wet handkerchief in the other. The man's a human waterfall.

Treating body odor

You attack this problem in three ways: by removing the offending bacteria with a bath or shower, inhibiting their growth with bacteriostat soaps and deodorants, or reducing the flow of perspiration by using antiperspirants and dressing sensibly.

Control over body odor obviously starts by **bathing daily** with plenty of soap to physically remove skin bacteria. Bathe in warm, not steaming, water. Rinse yourself thoroughly in clear water and towel briskly.

Deodorant soaps can be relatively effective because they inhibit the growth of odor-causing bacteria all over your body, but they don't really come to grips with the extreme conditions found under your arms and in your crotch where most of the smell comes from. Deodorant soaps contain ten to twenty times the bacteriostat in spray deodorants (between 1 and 2 per cent) because most of it gets washed away. What little remains after bathing rests on your skin and in your pores to inhibit bacteria growth.

Aerosol **deodorant sprays** are easy to use and, more importantly, very effective because this form enables you to apply neat bacteriostat directly onto your skin. Most sprays contain a combination of about .1 per cent bacteriostat, alcohol, which has a brief germ-killing effect, a propellent to force it out of the can, perfume, and sometimes a conditioning oil (about 2 per cent) to soothe your skin and replace any natural oil that may have been lost through using the spray.

Some men use deodorant sticks, which are basically alcoholic soap sticks containing a bacteriostat. Be sure to keep their caps tightly fixed against the air or they may shrink down to the size of a pencil.

How long does deodorant protection last? There's disagreement among manufacturers concerning the duration of deodorant effectiveness you can expect from using their products. This is probably due to formula variations and testing techniques, but your body also influences the effectiveness of a deodorant. If you normally sweat a lot or sweat more from exertion and climatic conditions, much of your deodorant will be washed away, thus reducing its effectiveness.

It's safe to say that under normal conditions, the average man can expect between twelve and twenty-four hours of protection from any well-formulated spray. If used in the morning and before going out in the evening, isn't that enough protection?

Are you immune to your deodorant? Some chemists believe that your body bacteria build up immunity to frequently used products, and this could be the case with deodorants. Others think it unlikely that deodorant-resistant strains of bacteria evolve, and from a practical standpoint, as most marketed deodorants contain the same few approved bacteriostats, they see little point in switching from the active ingredient in brand X to the same ingredient in brand Y.

As many effective deodorants exist today, the idea of alternating between them shouldn't worry you. I switch back and forth not only between deodorants but between antiperspirants, as conditions dictate.

Antiperspirants reduce the flow of sweat by either blocking up your pores or swelling the surrounding skin to shrink the size of the pore openings. Laboratories aren't exactly sure which of the two, or their combination, is responsible for restricting perspiration, but they know it works.

The most effective antiperspirants come in cream or roll-on form and, with continued use, can reduce sweat output by up to 40 per cent. Sprays reduce it about 20 per cent.

Cream formulations generally consist of water and fatty materials blended into a creamy base, perfume, and as much as 20 per cent of an aluminum compound, antiperspirant ingredient (often aluminum chlorohydrate), which is also a pretty effective deodorant. Thus antiperspirants control your body odor by reducing the quantity of sweat as well as inhibiting the growth of skin bacteria which feed on it. Although not really needed, some manufacturers add about .1 per cent of another bacteriostat to make sure of effective deodorant action and claim up to forty-eight hours of protection from this combination of ingredients.

The most popular spray antiperspirant formula is a dry one which doesn't have the watery feeling common to spray deodorants. Like creams, these sprays contain aluminum compounds as their major active ingredient, but in reduced quantities (usually between 3 and 5 per cent) because you spray it relatively undiluted onto your skin. Bacteriostats are generally, but not necessarily, added. The remainder of the formulation usually has a propellent, suspension agents, and perfume. Some manufacturers also add oils (about 5 per cent) to soothe your skin.

Is it dangerous to block the pores under your arms? This common question troubles many people. Although a long time ago, underarm sweat might have been needed to produce a "sexy" mating smell, it's not necessary today for any known body function. Blocking these pores represents no problem at all because there's so much skin area through which perspiration can escape; and besides, antiperspirants aren't 100 per cent effective, so some perspiration gets through.

Deodorants versus antiperspirants—which to use? As Gilbert and Sullivan wrote, "Let the punishment fit the crime." Keep both types on hand. Use a deodorant on those occasions when your activities and climatic conditions will be such that you don't expect to perspire much. Use an antiperspirant (spray or stronger cream) when the reverse is true, such as going dancing, to a crowded dinner, or vacationing in hot, humid climates. (Don't wear one while sunbathing.) Remember that nervousness in social and business situations can also increase perspiration, so take this into consideration when deciding which product to use.

The best defense for men with high fat content in their sweat is frequent washing coupled with an antiperspirant.

Antiperspirants have a drawback which you may have noticed—they can stain clothes. The aluminum compounds used in these products are also used in the dye industry to fix color to fabrics. The traces of these aluminum compounds left under the arms of your shirts and jackets pick up loose dye in wash water. Deodorants don't increase staining over normal expectations.

Experiment with different brands of each type. They can often react differently on your skin. You may need a formulation that contains some soothing skin oils or you may develop a minor allergy to various perfume ingredients or alcohol levels. You've got a lot to choose from.

CROTCH DEODORANTS

Because of the greater sensitivity of this area, deodorant formulations for the crotch must be more gentle than those used elsewhere. To my knowledge, antiperspirant aluminum salts aren't considered safe enough. These deodorants usually contain mild antiseptics and less alcohol than underarm products.

I have not seen sufficient test results to make concrete recommendations on the use and effectiveness of crotch deodorants at this time. Presumably an initial degree of deodorant protection can be obtained and, depending upon your evening activities, their light fragrance might prove more than a hidden asset.

One sure way of keeping crotch odor down is frequent washing and a daily change of underwear.

BODY ODOR AND CLOTHING

Under normal conditions, the average man loses about a pint of perspiration a day. This liquid has to go somewhere. Hopefully most of it will evaporate directly into the air as it would if you were in your bathing suit. What's left gets absorbed into your clothes where it produces a stale smell which quickly returns when they're worn again. Bearing this in mind, consider these five commonsense suggestions:

Change your clothes frequently. Certainly change your underwear and socks daily as well as shirts and other clothing that comes into direct contact with your moist skin.

Air your clothes. Allow your suits to dry and air before hanging them in the crowded closet with limited air circulation. Your wife may not like it, but hang them over the back of a chair overnight or, better still, use one of those free-standing "valets" on which you hang your clothes, rest your shoes, and unload your pockets. Keep your closet doors open as much as possible; what's the point of locking odor in? Let it out.

Dry-clean suits regularly to rid them of stale perspiration which starts smelling again when it comes in contact with your body warmth and moisture.

Be careful of synthetics. Many synthetic fabrics with a very high or 100 per cent man-made fiber content (like nylon) don't absorb perspiration as effectively as natural fibers. They can trap sweat against your skin where it turns sour and encourages bacteria growth. Cotton shirts and underwear and wool or cotton socks absorb sweat and "breathe" to aid air circulation and evaporation.

Dress sensibly. The weight and tightness of your clothing obviously affects your body temperature, perspiration, and your chance of body odor. Most homes, offices, cars, train, and planes are kept warm, if not too warm. Your only risk of chill these days comes from those brief periods when you run from one to the other. Dress for warmer interior environments in comfortable, lightweight clothes and put on a topcoat for the in-between times. In summer heat, wear loose-fitting clothes so air can circulate over as much of your skin's surface as possible.

Onion hands

The smell of onion has the unhappy ability of clinging tenaciously to the hands of the amateur or serious chef, and can be a real turn-off when you try to get "a little more comfortable" after your candlelight dinner for two. A very sexy cook once gave me this tip.

> Before peeling onions, wet your hands and gently rub a teaspoon of ordinary table salt over them. Don't rinse after that, just peel away. Replenish the salt when needed.

I can't explain why this works, but your hands hardly have a bit of onion smell when you finish. What little there may be will probably be masked when you splash after-shave on your face in preparation for the tryst.

FOOT ODOR

The causes

Like the body, smelly feet are caused by the growth of bacteria which thrive on perspiration. But unlike the body, your feet may have as many as 2,500 pores to the square inch; your back has only 400 to the inch. Also, snug-fitting shoes and socks inhibit air circulation and sweat evaporation which magnifies your problem.

It's normal for feet to have a "footy" smell, but not a strong odor. Foot odor runs the gamut from barely noticeable to the extreme pungent and offensive smell of bromidrosis, suffered by a relatively small percentage of men. Bromidrosis (caused by the interaction of *Bacterium fetidum* on the fat content of perspiration) can have serious social complications for its victims and should be tackled at once. So extreme is the odor that one expert told me he could recognize a man suffering from this condition the instant he walked into the office.

The treatment

Use the recommended treatments for various degrees of foot odor in the following chart. Select the one most pertinent to your problem or, if you have none, undertake good normal foot care. Carry out these treatments at least once a day; twice (morning and evening) if you have a serious problem. The regimen for bromidrosis should bring you relief in two to four weeks.

RECOMMENDED TREATMENTS FOR FOOT ODOR

TREATMENTS	*Normal care no odor*	*Some odor*	*Strong odor excessive perspiration*	*Extreme odor bromidrosis*
Wash your feet in warm, not hot, water and give them a good cold rinse.	x	x	x	
Bathe feet for 2 minutes in hot water and then ½ minute in cold. Alternate six times.				x

TREATMENTS	*Normal care no odor*	*Some odor*	*Strong odor excessive perspiration*	*Extreme odor bromidrosis*
Dry thoroughly, paying particular attention to between your toes.	x	x	x	x
Douse liberally with pure rubbing alcohol (diluted with water if your skin is, or becomes, inflamed) or spray on an alcoholic foot freshener. Allow to dry.	(For a tonic effect, or as a preventative after exposure to athlete's foot or other fungal disease.)			
Apply a foot deodorant.		x		
Apply a foot antiperspirant.			x	x
Dust your feet, especially between your toes, with a bacteriostat foot powder.	x	x	x	x
Change your socks daily.	x	x	x	x
Disinfect wool socks or boil cotton ones.				x
Air shoes nightly.	x	x	x	x
Change shoes on alternate days.	preferred	x	x	x
Disinfect shoes monthly.			if needed	x
Go barefoot or wear sandals when convenient.	x	x	x	x

CHAPTER 22

Drugs in Your Life

Are you addicted to drugs? Don't regard drugs as only those "evil" substances smuggled in from the East which other people, the social outcasts, take. You're forgetting the wife's tranquilizers, Aunt Edith's antidepressants, and your sleeping pills. They're all drugs, and so are those other pills and tablets you take to relieve major and minor or even imagined aches and pains. If you're not hooked on any of these, what about the caffeine stimulant in your coffee or tea, the nicotine in your cigarettes, and, of course, alcohol?

Dr. Joel Fort, in his study of a sophisticated American urban population, estimated that of any random selection of twenty adults, the chances are that fifteen drink moderately, two are problem drinkers, and one may well be an alcoholic. Two of the drinkers probably use marijuana, a couple take tranquilizers on doctor's orders, and one or two rely upon barbiturates for sleep. Three or four have taken amphetamines to stay awake or to help lose weight, and one may have taken acid or mescaline. About half the twenty continue to smoke after all warnings, and almost all drink caffeine in some form every day.

Many people have become overreliant on the legal drugs as cure-alls for everything from colds and aches to insomnia and anxiety, encouraging themselves to treat the effect rather than the cause. To my way of thinking, this is a negative way of approaching life. I believe more in mind over matter; that an optimistic and constructive attack on physical and mental problems is essential to a long, well-adjusted, and happy life.

The object of this chapter isn't to separate the good drugs from the bad—that's for you and your doctor to decide. It's simply to make you aware of what you're doing every time you pop a pill into your mouth and of the possible consequences of overdependence and abuse of drugs. In this case, ignorance is not bliss.

Finally, think of the drug environment that you may be creating for your children. Some recent studies suggest that children with parents who regularly take medicine in capsule form are three to ten times more likely to become drug abusers than children of parents who don't.

THE EFFECTS OF COMMON DRUGS ON YOUR MIND AND BODY

Aside from coffee, alcohol, and cigarettes, the types of legal drugs commonly used today under doctor's advice are tranquilizers, barbiturates (sleeping pills), and amphetamines (pep pills). The discussion of these drugs is based upon the short-term effects of taking the average, recommended dosages.

Tranquilizers

Tranquilizers generally relieve tension and anxiety and suppress aggressions and hallucinations associated with some forms of psychosis. They're often used in the treatment of alcoholism. You run a moderate risk of becoming psychologically and physically addicted to most tranquilizers (Thorazin appears to create no physical dependence).

The long-term effect of continued excessive use of tranquilizers could be destruction of your blood cells, jaundice, and, in extreme cases, death.

Barbiturates

Barbiturates are usually prescribed for insomnia and tension. They produce relaxation and a euphoric feeling of well-being. Your alertness and ability to co-ordinate decrease, leading to drowsiness and sleep.

During the first few weeks of barbiturate usage, you take less paradoxical sleep, but by the end of a month, your body has pretty much adjusted to the drugs and approaches a normal balance between the two types of sleep it needs. The risk of psychological and physical addiction to barbiturates is high. Increasing amounts are needed to produce the same effects as your body builds up its tolerance to them. When you withdraw from barbiturate usage after taking them for a month or so, it takes about five weeks before your sleep pattern between paradoxical and orthodox sleep returns to normal. During this process, you usually experience greater dream awareness and more nightmares.

Amphetamines

Amphetamines increase your alertness and excitation and give you a feeling of euphoria. They're used to overcome depression and excessive fatigue and to fight obesity by decreasing your appetite.

Although the risk of becoming psychologically dependent on amphetamines is high, physical addiction appears to be nil. Your body, however, does build up its tolerance to the drugs, necessitating larger dosages as you continue their use. Some of the long-term effects of excessive amphetamine usage are insomnia, excitability, psychosis, malnutrition, and skin disorders. Withdrawal from the drugs can create a violent reaction to insomnia and often irrational depression.

If barbiturates and amphetamines have been used together, withdrawal may take as long as two months before your normal sleeping pattern can be restored. This time closely approximates the time needed for your brain to renew and reprogram its cells.

Warning

Beware of buying drugs on the illicit market. Unfortunately, there's no quality control over illicit drug sales of barbiturates, amphetamines, marijuana, hashish, mescaline, and others. American studies show between 50 and 70 per cent of drugs sold illegally contain something other than advertised. These adulterating substances can be dangerous if not deadly. Also, the strength of these drugs can vary greatly, making it difficult to anticipate the intensity of their effects. For example, LSD is often put up in amounts three times too strong for the casual user to handle, and deaths result from heroin overdoses caused by shots with unexpectedly high drug content.

Coffee and tea

Both coffee and tea contain the drug caffeine, which stimulates your nervous system to make you feel more awake and encourages activity and conversation. (This could explain the current revival of the coffee houses so popular in the seventeenth and eighteenth centuries with literary men.) As the effect wears off, you may feel a mild depression and the consequent need for another pick-me-up cup. This can lead to coffee addiction.

Men differ in their sensitivity to caffeine, but the average man should be able to drink three to four cups of coffee a day without ill effects. Depending upon your reaction, too much caffeine may bring on headache, insomnia, nausea, disturbed vision, shakiness, giddiness, irritability, and anxiety feelings.

If you notice any of these symptoms, consider switching your current brand of coffee to a decaffeinated one, or drink tea, which has about half the caffeine content per cup. For you connoisseurs, China tea is said to contain less caffeine than Indian tea.

ALCOHOL—HOW TO DRINK WITHOUT PAIN

While liquor, beer, and wine can produce relaxation and euphoria, they can also produce depression, decreased alertness, and the dreaded hangover.

You suffer hangovers when your liver, one of your most effective cleansing organs, has been so overloaded with alcohol that it becomes sluggish and can't filter your blood completely. The impurities remaining in your blood cause the headache and tired, washed-out feeling generally associated with hangovers. Also, your stomach can be irritated by alcohol and usually doesn't want to know about anything the next day.

Be gentle with your woman the morning after; she'll probably suffer a worse hangover than you if she tried to keep up with you last night. Being smaller, women usually have smaller livers than men. Thus on a drink-for-drink basis, they overload their livers faster and more severely than men.

The unique quality of each type of spirit comes from varied amounts and combinations of its flavor constituents called congeners. They also may be responsible for the difference in the quality of the hangover each type gives. Experienced drinkers say gin and vodka lead to the mildest hangovers (their congener content is about 0.04 per cent and 0.01 per cent respectively). Bourbon (containing the most congeners, 0.31 per cent) and brandy (0.24 per cent) result in the most severe hangovers. Even though its congener level is very low, many people rate a beer hangover worst of all.

How to avoid a hangover: The sanest way to drink is to do it with your meals. A double whiskey before dinner, several glasses of wine during the meal, and the relaxed sipping of a large, and good, brandy afterward should see you happily through the evening with no regrets the next day. The equivalent amount of alcohol taken in the form of spirits at a cocktail party (approximately four double something-or-others) can usually get Mr. Average pretty high or drunk for a few hours, and present him with a hangover. It has also been found that alcohol, when drunk under quiet and relaxed conditions in fresh air, has less intoxicating and hangover effects than when consumed surrounded by blaring music, frantic cocktail chatter, and cigarette smoke.

Defend yourself against hangovers by drinking a glass of water for every whiskey and soda, gin and tonic, martini, or whatever. This dilutes the alcohol mixture heading for your liver. If you've had a lot to drink, two or three cups of black coffee taken while the alcohol is still sloshing about in your stomach may help prevent or lessen a hangover. The coffee stimulates your groggy nervous system and spreads the absorption of alcohol into your blood over a longer period of time.

The better the condition of your liver, the better it will function to filter out hangover-producing impurities from your blood. So it stands to reason that by keeping your body and its organs in good over-all health, you'll help your liver cope more effectively with any excess of alcohol you pour through it from time to time.

Hangover remedies: The different hangover "cures" that you'll come across during your lifetime will probably fill an encyclopedia. Every barman has his favorite. I approached the following "morning after" remedy scientifically with the aid of a research chemist. The three areas of hangover discomfort have been taken into account: headache, an irritated and upset stomach, and the general malaise and fatigue.

> In a large glass, beat two egg yolks (to line your stomach), add the juice of a lemon or lime (for flavor and vitamin C), fill the glass with cold soda or tonic water (the fizz soothes your stomach), add two soluble aspirins (for headache pain) and a teaspoon of sugar (to speed absorption and for energy).

This combination makes a cool, soothing, and rather bland-tasting brew, which goes down very well first thing in the morning.

If you reject this solution, at least follow its principles:

- Force yourself to eat a good breakfast to take the raw edge out of your stomach.
- Only then should you take your aspirin or aspirin-based pain killers. Aspirin has an irritating effect on your stomach, particularly when it's empty and already irritated by alcohol. Put a lining down first.
- Add sugar to your coffee or tea and drink sweetened fruit juice to build up your blood sugar level as fast as possible.
- Sip a fizzy drink from time to time to help settle and soothe your stomach.

Many doctors now agree that the best cure for a hangover is another drink. During the hangover, your nervous system is very sluggish and its reactions can be improved with another jolt of alcohol, but only until that jolt is burned up. The bloody mary, with its low congener vodka base, ranks high here. Just remember, however, you're only postponing the first hangover while building up to a worse one later on in the day. You've got to stop the cycle sometime.

Smoke sensibly

If you're still smoking cigarettes after all the warnings, I'm sure nothing this book can say will alter your mind. I offer only two bits of advice on the subject. If you must smoke, then smoke the brands lowest in harmful nicotine and tars. You can get this information easily from consumer publications or government health sources.

If you really want to stop smoking but find it terribly hard, you might try the method I used to break the habit gradually and painlessly. Just purchase the brand of cigarette you hate the most and make a reasonable effort to smoke only when you feel a strong desire to do so. As I no longer enjoyed the taste and sensation of smoking, I found myself lighting fewer cigarettes and inhaling less of each. After a few months, my daily intake was down so low that stopping all together was very easy and hardly noticed.

A GOOD USE FOR CIGARETTES

For you confirmed smokers who are also keen gardeners, here's your chance to combine your vice with your hobby: Make an insecticide from your old filter tips.

The nicotine in tobacco is a deadly poison. While smoking, it becomes concentrated in the filters of your cigarettes. Simmer two ounces of filter tips in a quart of water for half an hour, replacing the water as it boils away. Strain the clear brown liquid through a fine mesh like an old nylon stocking. Dilute with four quarts of cold water to spray tough insects like caterpillars, or with six quarts to kill those like aphids. Make up the mixture as required and *keep it away from children.*

This recipe was taken from the *Sunday Times* in London one spring, just in time for the bug season.

Chapter 23

Summary: Improving Your Virility, Fitness, and Looks

Why should one identical twin look and act thirty-five, and the other fifty?

You've seen how your body's defense systems gradually begin to falter and its ability to repair itself lessens with age. With its declining resources, your body must act with utmost economy, devoting primary attention to the essentials of staying alive; what's left over goes toward maintaining the attractiveness and youthful looks of the nonessentials like your hair and skin.

Therefore, like the younger-looking twin, make every effort to keep your mind and body in shape and protect them from undue stress, illness, and injury, which can drain their resources and prematurely wear you out. The more help you give it, the longer your body will be able to keep living and looking the way you want it to.

Put it all together. Draw on the previous chapters for the many ways to improve your virility, fitness, and looks. The earlier you start, the better.

THINK POSITIVE

Liza Minnelli once turned on a rather morbid interviewer who tried to probe into the "darker side" of her relationship with her mother, Judy Garland. She flashed out with, "Who cares about the darker side—screw the darker side! Life's marvelous, it's happening now, let's talk about that." With an approach to life like this, I'm sure Ms. Minnelli will live a long, youthful, and happy life.

A recent study of sixty-to-ninety-four-year-olds found that morale and work satisfaction were better predicators of long life than physical fitness, smoking history, nutritional status, or parental age at death. It's in your mind.

Your approach to life should be optimistic, interested, and active. Keep your mind receptive and stimulated by seeking new adventures and experiences. Don't pontificate on the past, but look to the future.

Create the right environment in which to live and work. Keep it stimulating, but calm, secure, and happy. Eliminate people and things that irritate you. Don't be a guilt-ridden adrenaline addict, but enjoy leisure time and relaxation. Manage your business life effectively. Delegate responsibility. Don't exhaust your mind and body with needless overwork and don't identify personally with all the problems around you. As we said, play it cool.

LIVE YOUNG

Keep your body well fueled and oiled and in as good repair as possible so it can run efficiently and hold on to its youthful appearance longer.

Eat a balanced diet to give a healthy body all the raw materials it needs to function at peak efficiency. No crash diets unless under your doctor's supervision. Keep nonessential carbohydrate intake low for weight control and to stop damage to your teeth and gums.

Control your weight. Try to get back (or keep) the slim weight of your university days. Obesity puts great wear and tear on your body's support systems, aside from not looking very good on you.

Stay physically fit to help keep your body structure strong and flexible and your respiratory and cardiovascular systems functioning properly. If you let them run down, you'll force yourself into a more limited life pattern.

- Stretch your muscles and joints every day to keep them limber.
- Exercise by walking more and climbing stairs. Enter into sports activities. Swim, play tennis, or do some cardiovascular calisthenics.
- Keep your supporting back and abdominal muscles strong and your posture good. It may eliminate much pain and disability later on.
- For a youthful appearance, exercise your chin and throat muscles to keep them firm and, again, keep that stomach flat.
- Stay out of sauna and steam rooms.

Get enough sleep to enable your brain and body to recuperate and to increase your resistance to illness.

Head off serious illness and disease. The best way to spend money is to stop illness before it takes hold and knocks the hell out of your system. Have regular medical checkups.

Use alcohol in moderation for enjoyment and to relax yourself. Remember that as you age, your liver copes less effectively with alcohol and can be seriously damaged by continued excesses.

Stop smoking, primarily because of its connection with cancer and heart problems, but also because there's some evidence that it can age your skin.

Hold on to your virility by keeping in good physical condition and maintaining an active and adventurous sex life. If you're over sixty and feel the need for a boost, talk with your doctor about hormone injections and implants.

LOOK BETTER

Your mind and body go hand in hand. Help maintain the youthful appearance of your body's outer shell to stimulate a youthful outlook on life. Supplement your body's waning natural functions, protect it from hostile environments, and groom and restore it to look more attractive.

Keep your skin from aging as much as possible by fighting dryness and wrinkles. Spend less time in your shower or bath if you've got dry skin, and go easy on soap and hot water. Follow the right cleansing regimen for your face and use a moisturizer. When needed, rub on a lotion or oil to help keep your body skin soft and smooth.

Avoid excessive exposure to the sun which can toughen and age your skin and damage your hair. Protect your eyes with the proper sunglasses.

Consider cosmetic plastic surgery to remove bags and wrinkles around your eyes or to tighten up your facial muscles and skin. This is one of the most effective and dramatic ways of keeping youthful in both spirit and looks. Also consider correcting any part of your bone structure that you and your doctor feel detracts from your appearance.

Keep healthy hair and scalp with regular shampooing (use dandruff remedies if needed) and care. Make sure you have a good comb which isn't damaging your hair, and avoid using a brush and rough massage.

A youthful hairstyle for you may not necessarily be the one that young people wear. A shorter style is usually more attractive and flattering to older men. Consider restoring the natural color to graying hair and using transplants or hairpieces to replace lost hair.

Remove superfluous hair which is unflattering to you. Pluck hair growing on your nose and trim hair growing out of your nose, ears, and between your eyebrows. In other words, tidy yourself up.

Keep your teeth and gums looking clean and healthy. Restorations should be invisible to the eye. Use crowns, bridges, or dentures to eliminate discolored, uneven teeth and to fill obvious gaps. Give yourself an attractive smile.

Protect your hands from drying and hostile environments and rub in a natural oil once a day. Keep your **fingernails well groomed** and remove any age ridges as they appear. Above all, keep your cuticles smooth and lifted.

Go barefoot or wear exercise sandals when practical. Periodically **groom your toenails** and stop the growth of uncomfortable corns and thick calluses by wearing properly fitted shoes.

There are many very simple things you can do to keep your body and mind feeling and looking great. We're all on this earth such a short time. Let's make the most of it and live one hell of a good time.

Appendix I

How to Buy and Use Grooming Aids; What Ones to Beware

How to buy grooming preparations

When choosing a straightforward after-shave lotion to splash on your face, you're basically buying a male perfume. Fragrance must be your prime concern and depends upon your taste and that of your woman. Don't just sniff from the bottle; smell it on your skin before making a final selection.

Other grooming preparations like shampoos, deodorants, and skin creams need more thought because they must do more than just smell nice. First, decide why you're buying a particular type of product, its purpose, and what short- and long-term effects you want from it. Is it to clean your hair, make it more manageable, and/or inhibit dandruff? Do you want a simple moisturizing cream or one that doubles as a fragrance or has cosmetic properties to make your skin look tan? Once you've made up your mind, look for the product that best suits your needs.

Read very carefully the claims made for preparations by their manufacturers. Although they tend to guild the emotional lily a bit, by law they must tell the truth. Be guided by the *actual* promised benefits, not the *implied* ones. Ask the experts—your doctor, dermatologist, or pharmacist—for their recommendations. Keep your eyes open for reports from consumer testing organizations like *Which?* and *Consumers' Report*.

What about cost?

The cost of a product bears little relation to its effectiveness. Much of the price of a grooming preparation lies in its perfume and chic packaging. A shampoo or cleansing cream bought in a supermarket may be just as beneficial, if not more so, as those gift-wrapped in Mayfair or on Park Avenue.

Buy the smallest size of a new preparation to see how you like it. If you're satisfied that it lives up to its promises and you have no allergic reaction to it, move on to the larger economy sizes; but first make sure they are, in fact, an economy.

Take advantage of your favorite brands' "price-off" promotions and stock up on those you normally use a lot, like bar soaps, toothpastes, deodorants. You'll not only save money, but can generally be sure they haven't been sitting on store shelves a long time.

Where to buy?

Because of the limited life of many fragrances, I usually buy my grooming preparations in large stores or shops that have a fast turnover in these types of products. In this way, the time between the manufacture of a preparation and your bathroom cabinet will be minimal and you have time to use it up long before the fragrance or formulation goes off.

How to use them

Obviously, follow the directions exactly, and don't over- or underuse them. Manufacturers base their claims and promises on the recommended usage of their preparations, not on your whims. Make sure you don't use them in the wrong sequence so they nullify the effects of each other. Also, it's wasteful and unnecessary to use several preparations at the same time that duplicate one another's functions.

Keep fragrances and grooming preparations at their peak levels of effectiveness by protecting them from sunlight and extreme temperatures. (Sixty degrees Fahrenheit is a good average temperature.) Also, keep them away from air which will oxidize their natural ingredients and help put them off. Screw or snap lids firmly in place and allow as little air space to develop in bottles as possible. Pour half-full bottles of after-shave lotions into smaller ones, or keep adding transparent glass marbles to keep the liquid level high. (That's what many laboratories do.) Once open, use up a fragrance or preparation as quickly as practical and then open another. Don't keep a wide variety going at any one time, no matter how many you got for Christmas.

Fragrances

Almost every grooming preparation a man uses contains some fragrance. Current tastes run more to the sophisticated scents of real perfumes made on the French line—lighter, with more staying power.

Men's fragrances, like perfume, generally consist of a complicated blending and maturation of citron, floral, or other highly scented oils and chemical synthetics with an animal fixative which makes the scent stick and last on your skin. These fixatives are often repulsive: ambergris (part of a sperm whale's stomach lining), castoreum (perineal glands of beavers), or substances from the genital regions of the southern Asian and African civet and the male musk deer. They're extremely expensive, but fortunately only a very little goes a long way.

Why does a fragrance change?

The fragrance of any one brand is affected by the particular pH level of your skin, which can vary with tension, diet, and age. That's why you should smell a perfume on your skin before buying it.

Also, the life of fragrances usually averages about a year from the date of manufacture before they start going off. The scent of one widely used after-shave lotion and body perfume must mature for sixteen days before bottling, after which it continues to mature for a further six months before reaching its peak. The fragrance level stays constant for the next six months and then gradually declines and starts going sour.

Expect the fragrance of your favorite brands to be slightly different if put in aerosol form. Standard formulations must usually be adapted to disguise the odor of aerosol propellants.

What products to beware?

I believe it's safe to say there's no product manufactured to which someone isn't allergic. Some men have broken out in rashes from sleeping next to the dyed hair of their wives. Sooner or later you may run into this problem from a grooming preparation or you may become temporarily photosensitive because of the reaction of some drug or toiletry to the sun. If and when your skin shows sensitivity, carefully review every product you're using with your doctor and try to find and eliminate the offender.

There are some preparations and ingredients that you should avoid or use with extreme care:

> **Hair-coloring products** should be tested on your skin (patch tests) for allergic reactions to their dyes before use. *Keep them away from your eyes.*
>
> Use **aerosol hair sprays** carefully. Don't risk fire or explosion by smoking when applying them. Keep your eyes closed and hold your breath. If inhaled, some aerosols can give you a

mild "high," but also may muck up your lungs and have harmful effects on your heart.

Talcum powder: Make sure there's no dangerous asbestos in the formulation you use. Also, don't apply a body talc to your feet instead of special foot powders. The fineness of some body talcs may clog the pores of your feet.

Hexachlorophene, the germ killer once found in many deodorants, has been banned as dangerous in Germany and its use severely restricted in the United States and France. It was the suspected cause of death of twenty-eight babies who were exposed to excessive amounts of it in a talcum powder.

Deodorants and antiperspirants: If you plan extensive sunbathing, play safe and don't apply these products to your skin before stripping off. They might encourage a photosensitive reaction in your skin. The same applies to the use of the more concentrated forms of fragrance or perfume.

Bubble bath and bath foams often contain detergents which may be drying to your skin. If used, I suggest you apply a little body oil afterward unless you have naturally oily skin.

Enzyme products used for cleaning should be thoroughly rinsed off your skin. So, too, should soaps and detergents.

Hormone products: Men should be very wary about using any products containing estrogens because of the possible feminizing effects of overdoses in their systems. And besides, tests indicate hormones in preparations sold without a doctor's prescription have no visible benefits for skin over those received from the base product. (One chemist who took estrogens in an experiment to inhibit balding developed breasts. It was some time before both his chest and ego got back to normal.)

Deceptive containers in the form of attractive toys or looking as if they could hold edible substances can be a danger to children as well as careless adults. Toiletries work best on, not in, your body.

APPENDIX 2

The Low-Carbohydrate Diet for Men

This diet* will give you appetizing meals and fill you up, and yet it contains only about 1,200 calories a day—less than half the normal intake for men. You'll eat well while growing thin.

EAT THREE MEALS A DAY

Every day you must eat:

- Breakfast
- One light meal *plus* fruit or a sweet dessert
- One main meal *plus* fruit or a sweet dessert

* This recommended diet was developed by the nutritionists of the Energen Foods Company. Only minor adjustments have been made.

With these meals you may have a daily allowance of the following foods (the quantities of any of these foods used in cooking must be deducted from your allowance):

1½ cups of milk
1 tablespoon of butter or margarine
2 slices of bread or six diet crackers or crispbreads (like Ry Krisp or Energen Crispbreads).
3 level teaspoons of low-sugar diet jam or marmalade

Unrestricted food: You can eat reasonable portions (no need to measure) of the "unrestricted foods" listed at the end of this section with your meals to make them more filling and interesting. But remember, even the unrestricted foods contain calories, so don't go overboard.

Restricted foods: Avoid all "restricted foods" listed at the end of this section except those recommended exceptions.

Breakfasts

Choose from:

1 small glass (4 oz.) of unsweetened fruit juice

or

1 portion of fruit, fresh or stewed, with the addition of a nonsugar sweetener after cooking if desired

or

1 cup (¾ oz.) of a nonsugared, starch-reduced, or high-protein cold cereal

Plus any ONE of the following:

1 egg (boiled, poached, baked, scrambled, or in an omelet)

or

1 lean strip of bacon (broiled or baked)

or

1 oz. of lean cold ham

or

3 oz. white fish (broiled, baked, or poached) or smoked haddock

or

1 small kipper or herring (broiled, poached, or baked)

Plus the following:

Broiled or baked tomatoes or mushrooms,
Toast or crispbread with butter or margarine and low-sugar diet jam or marmalade from your allowance, and
Tea or coffee with milk from your allowance, with nonsugar sweetener if desired

Main Meals

Portion weights for lean, uncooked meat off the bone are 4 oz. (¼ pound). Portion weights for uncooked fish are 8 oz. (½ pound).

- Roast meat or poultry and bean sprouts
- Braised chicken and carrots or white cabbage
- Boiled Tongue with Orange Sauce* and leeks or Brussels sprouts
- Poached smoked haddock and spinach
- Broiled ham and tomato with green beans
- Boiled ham and green vegetables
- Lamb chops and cabbage or celery
- Cod or Haddock Cheese Delight* and tomatoes or cucumbers
- Stuffed pepper or savory mince and broccoli or turnips
- Broiled or braised liver and endive or cauliflower
  (Liver is a particularly rich source of many nutrients, so try to eat it at least once a week.)
- Boiled beef and carrots with braised onions

* Recipes follow at the end of this section.

- Baked or broiled mackerel with baked tomatoes and squash or Brussels sprouts
- Steak and Kidney Hot Pot* and sea kale or cabbage
- Mixed grill or Kebabs* and cabbage or spinach
- Baked Meat Loaf* and braised celery or leeks
- Broiled lamb or pork chop and stewed red cabbage and apple, or Brussels sprouts
- Broiled or baked herring and grated raw cabbage and onion with yogurt, or broiled tomato
- Stewed veal or tripe and cauliflower or green beans

Light Meals

Portion weights for lean, uncooked meat off the bone are 3 oz. Portion weights for uncooked fish are 6 oz.

- Canned salmon and cucumber and watercress
- Cold cooked chicken or broiled chicken and lettuce
- Bacon and egg cooked together in frypan and lettuce, or broiled bacon, hard-boiled egg, and lettuce
- Welsh rarebit on toast or crispbreads (from your allowance) and broiled tomatoes
- Cold ham or jellied veal and cold fresh beans and dressing
- Stuffed hard-boiled egg, the yolk mixed with anchovy paste or grated cheese, and lettuce or endive
- Sardines, drained of oil, and lettuce and tomato
- Boiled ham or corned beef and sliced tomato and chicory salad
- Broiled or baked cod roe and tomato and watercress salad
- Mushroom, shrimp, or Cheese Omelet* and lettuce and tomato
- Cheese and a shrimp salad
- Poached egg on spinach
- Ham and a watercress and orange salad

- Pickled, broiled, or baked herring and a chopped celery, apple, and green pepper salad
- Crisped Chicken* and green salad
- Cheese soufflé and baked tomatoes
- Baked Hamburgers* and broiled tomatoes or cold sliced tomatoes and onions
- Tongue or beef Open Sandwiches*

Sweet Desserts

- Apple Crunch*
- Fruit gelatin (Jell-O)
- Baked apple, stuffed with 1 teaspoon of low-sugar diet jam
- Junket
- Plain yogurt with 1 teaspoon of low-sugar diet jam
- Egg custard
- Fresh fruit salad
- Lemon mousse
- Fruit canned in water (not sugar syrup)
- Baked whole oranges
- Baked peaches or pears
- Apricot and Orange Mousse*
- Rhubarb with crunch topping
- 1 oz. of cheese and crispbreads (from your allowance)

Fruits

• Fresh or baked apple	1 medium
• Applesauce (unsweetened)	1½ cups
• Fresh apricots	3 to 4 medium
• Fresh blackberries	1 cup
• Fresh cherries	1 cup
• Fresh plums	2 medium
• Stewed plums (unsweetened)	½ cup

• Orange	1 medium
• Tangerines	2 medium
• Fresh peach	1 large
• Fresh pear	1 small
• Stewed pears (unsweetened)	½ cup
• Fresh pineapple	1 medium slice
• Fresh strawberries	1 cup
• Fresh raspberries	1 cup

Unrestricted Foods

You may eat as much as you like of the following foods. Add them to the recommended meals for variety and interest.

Fruit: grapefruit, melon, rhubarb, lemon

Vegetables: cauliflower, spinach, french beans, cabbage, asparagus, squash, bean sprouts

Salads and garnishings: lettuce, watercress, tomatoes, mushrooms, parsley, mixed herbs, spices

Special salad dressings: You can make appetizing salad dressings with any of the following: vinegar, lemon juice, salt, pepper, and herbs such as dill, marjoram, or chopped parsley. Make an excellent thick, creamy dressing with a little yogurt, dill, grated onion, seasoning, a little hot water, and a nonsugar sweetener.

Drinks: black coffee, tea, unsweetened soda water, clear soup, vegetable and meat extracts or concentrates

Restricted Foods

Cut out all of the following foods from your diet.

Flour and all foods made from flour: cakes, pastry, puddings, spaghetti, macaroni, and biscuits, bread (except that on your allowance)

Cereal foods, oatmeal, rice, cornstarch and custard powder, cold breakfast cereals other than that in the diet breakfast.

Sugar, honey, glucose, syrup, ordinary jams and marmalades

Thick soups, thick sauces, soup mixes, and gravies

All fried foods, sausages, and cooking oils

Mayonnaise, salad dressings (except those recommended), chutney, and sweet pickles

Ice cream and cream

Nuts, peanut butter, and coconuts

Vegetables: potatoes, beets, parnsips, peas, lentils, lima or broad beans, butter beans, and baked beans

Dried and canned fruits, including those canned in syrup and sorbitol, raisins, sultanas, currants

Candy, sweets, and chocolate, including "diabetic" chocolate made with sorbitol

Chocolate and malted drinks

Condensed and evaporated milk

Cordials and bottled fruit juices, still or sparkling (sweetened with sorbitol), tonic water, canned lemonade, and soft drinks

Alcohol

Each large whiskey or gin or bottle of beer will give you the equivalent in calories of about a half pound of potatoes. You should therefore be careful about alcohol while reducing your weight. Dry white wine is your best bet if you want to go on being the life of the party.

Fitting in with the Family:

The Main Meals outlined above have been planned to do away with tiresome special cooking. Vegetables should be plain boiled, then when you slimmers have been served, the rest of the family can add their butter and sauces. Meat and fish should be cooked simply, without oils and other fattening fixings. Stewed fruits can be sweetened after cooking to fit both this diet and the tastes of the nonslimmers.

DIET RECIPES

Steak and Kidney Hot Pot

(*serves 4*)

Cooking time 1½–2 hours

¾ pound diced stewing beef
¼ pound lamb or pork kidneys, cored and diced
3 cups water
1 beef bouillon cube
1 large onion, chopped
2 carrots, peeled and sliced
2 celery ribs, chopped
2 leeks, sliced
1 tablespoon tomato puree
Salt and pepper

Place beef and kidney in pan with water. Bring to a boil slowly and skim fat from surface. Add bouillon cube, onion, carrots, and celery. Simmer for 1 hour. Add leeks to pan and continue to simmer for approximately ½ hour or until meat is tender. Stir in tomato puree. Season to taste with salt and pepper.

Baked Meat Loaf

(*serves 4*)

Cooking time: 35–40 minutes

½ pound pork liver, minced or finely chopped
½ pound lean beef, minced
1 tablespoon finely chopped green pepper
1 8-ounce can tomatoes
1 lightly beaten egg
Salt and pepper
1 teaspoon mixed herbs
1 tablespoon tomato puree

Preheat oven to 350°. Combine all the ingredients except the tomato puree. Grease a 9″ by 5″ loaf pan lightly and line with grease-proof paper. Transfer mixture to pan and bake. Remove from oven and drain off the liquid. Add tomato puree to the liquid and bring to a boil. Serve this hot sauce with the meat loaf.

Boiled Tongue with Orange Sauce

(*serves 4*)

Cooking time: 1½ hours plus 15–20 minutes

1 pound lamb or beef tongue
1 teaspoon low-sugar diet marmalade
Juice of 1 orange

Soak tongue in cold water for 2 hours. Then boil for 1½ hours, allow to cool, and remove skin and bones and trim. Preheat oven to 350°. Blend marmalade with orange juice. Slice tongue and arrange in baking dish. Pour sauce over, cover and place in oven for 15–20 minutes.

Kebabs

(*serves 4*)

Cooking time: approximately 10 minutes

1 onion, quartered
1 green pepper, cored and sliced
½ pound rump steak, cubed
¼ pound liver, diced
¼ pound lean bacon
¼ pound quartered tomatoes
1 3½-ounce can whole mushrooms

Place onion and pepper in boiling salted water for 2–3 minutes. Drain. Place pieces of steak, liver, and bacon rolls on 4 large skewers alternating with vegetable pieces. Broil for 10 minutes, turning frequently. Serve on a bed of cooked cabbage.

Cod or Haddock Cheese Delight

(*serves 1*)

Cooking time: 8–10 minutes

¼ pound fresh haddock or cod fillet
Melted butter
2 tablespoons grated cheddar cheese
1 teaspoon chopped parsley

Skin the fillet of haddock and wipe. Brush with a little melted butter and broil. Sprinkle with the grated cheese when fish is nearly cooked. Broil for a few minutes more, until the cheese has melted and browned slightly. Sprinkle with chopped parsley before serving.

Baked Hamburgers

(*serves 4*)

Cooking time: 30 minutes

1 pound lean beef, minced
2 tablespoons finely chopped onion
1 tablespoon finely chopped parsley
1 egg, lightly beaten
Salt and pepper
1 teaspoon dry mustard
Few drops Worcestershire sauce
1⅓ cups crushed corn or wheat flakes

Preheat oven to 375°. Combine all the ingredients except the corn or wheat flakes and mix thoroughly. Form mixture into eight patties and flatten. Roll each patty in the flakes. Enclose in foil and bake.

Crisped Chicken

(*serves 1*)

Cooking time: 25–30 minutes

1 large chicken drumstick or a small second joint
1 tablespoon milk
Salt and pepper
⅓ cup crushed corn or wheat flakes

Preheat oven to 375°. Rinse chicken and brush with milk. Season with salt and pepper and roll or dip in the corn or wheat flakes. Place in oven. Serve hot or cold with salad. (Note: This can be cooked while the oven is in use for other things.)

Cheese Omelet

(*serves 1*)

1 large egg, beaten
1 tablespoon water
Salt and pepper
½ tablespoon butter or margarine
2 tablespoons grated cheese

Mix egg, water, and seasoning together thoroughly with a whisk. Melt butter in frying pan. Increase heat and pour mixture into the pan. Stroke mixture toward the center until the surface is softly set. Sprinkle the cheese over the surface and fold the edges toward the center. Tilt the pan, allowing omelet to roll over onto serving platter.

Open Sandwiches

(*serves 1*)

½ tablespoon butter
2 crispbreads or diet crackers
Lettuce leaves
1 slice cooked beef (1 ounce)
1 thin slice cheese (¼ ounce)
1 tomato, sliced
Watercress
Radish slices

Spread butter lightly on crispbreads. Arrange lettuce on both. Top one with beef, the other with cheese. Garnish each with tomato, watercress, and radish slices.

Apple Crunch

(*serves 4*)

Cooking time: 15–20 minutes

1 pound cooking apples, peeled, cored, and sliced
2 tablespoons water
6–8 nonsugar sweetener tablets
1½ tablespoons margarine or butter
2 cups corn or wheat flakes

Preheat oven to 400°. Cook apples gently with water in covered pan for approximately 10 minutes. Beat until soft and pureed. Dissolve sweetener tablets in apple mixture and transfer to oven-proof dish. Melt margarine or butter in pan, remove from heat, and fold in flakes. Spread this topping evenly over apples. Place in oven until topping is evenly browned. Serve hot. (Note: Rhubarb may be used instead of apples.)

Apricot and Orange Mousse

(*serves 4*)

4 tablespoons dried milk
½ cup cold water
2 teaspoons gelatin
1 tablespoon boiling water
⅜ cup (3 fluid ounces) low-sugar diet apricot jam
Grated rind of 1 orange
1 orange, peeled and cut into pieces

Sprinkle the dried milk onto cold water and whisk until soft peaks form. Dissolve gelatin in boiling water. Mix in jam. Grate rind into whisked milk and fold in gelatin mixture and orange pieces. Pour into individual glasses and chill until set.

Appendix 3

Food Composition Tables

Foods	*Calories in 100 grams**	*Calories per portion*	*Approximate size of portion*	*Protein grams*	*Fat grams*	*Carbohydrate grams*
Dairy Produce						
Cheese						
Camembert	308	88	1 oz.	7	7	—
Cheddar	420	120	1 oz.	7	10	—
Cheshire	385	110	1 oz.	7	9	—
cottage (creamed)	106	30	1 oz.	4	1	1
cottage (uncreamed)	86	25	1 oz.	5	—†	1

SOURCE: U. S. Department of Agriculture Handbook. No. 8 and "The Composition of Foods" (Her Majesty's Stationery Office, 1969).

* Based upon the edible portions of each food.

† Less than one gram of protein, fat, or carbohydrate. (U. S. Government Printing Office).

Foods	Calories in 100 grams*	Calories per portion	Approximate size of portion	Protein grams	Fat grams	Carbohydrate grams
cream	375	107	1 oz.	2	12	—
Danish blue	360	103	1 oz.	7	8	—
Edam	308	88	1 oz.	7	7	—
Gorgonzola	392	112	1 oz.	7	9	—
Gouda	336	96	1 oz.	6	8	—
Gruyère	462	132	1 oz.	11	10	—
Parmesan	413	118	1 oz.	10	9	1
processed	371	106	1 oz.	7	9	—
Stilton	473	135	1 oz.	7	11	—
Swiss	355	100	1 oz.	8	8	—
Cocoa	97	250	1 cup	10	12	27
Cream						
light						
(coffee)	211	500	1 cup	8	52	11
heavy						
(whipping)	352	840	1 cup	5	98	7
Eggs						
cooked in shell	160	160	2 eggs	13	12	1
Ice Cream						
(12% fat)	207	390	1 cup	8	25	41
Ices, water	78	148	1 cup	1	—	60
Milk						
whole	66	330	1 pt.	18	19	25
skim	36	180	1 pt.	18	1	26
evaporated						
(unsweetened)	137	345	1 cup	16	—	24
malted	104	260	1 cup	12	11	30
Yogurt						
skimmed milk	50	125	1 cup	9	4	13
whole milk	62	155	1 cup	8	9	12

Foods	*Calories in 100 grams**	*Calories per portion*	*Approximate size of portion*	*Protein grams*	*Fat grams*	*Carbohydrate grams*
Oils, Fats, and Shortenings						
Butter	716	800	½ cup	—	90	1
	716	100	1 tbs.	—	11	—
Cooking oils	884	1000	½ cup	—	112	—
	884	125	1 tbs.	—	14	—
Dressings						
French	410	60	1 tbs.	—	6	2
Thousand Islands	502	75	1 tbs.	—	8	1
Lard	902	992	½ cup	—	110	—
Margarine	720	806	½ cup	—	91	—
Mayonnaise	718	110	1 tbs.	—	12	—
Fish and Seafoods						
Bass						
sea (baked and stuffed)	259	259	3½ oz.	16	16	11
striped (oven-fried)	196	196	3½ oz.	22	9	7
Caviar						
pressed sturgeon	316	90	1 oz.	10	4	3
Clams						
raw (soft meat only)	82	82	6 or 7 3½ oz.	14	2	1
Cod (boiled)	170	170	3½ oz.	29	5	—

Foods	*Calories in 100 grams**	*Calories per portion*	*Approximate size of portion*	*Protein grams*	*Fat grams*	*Carbohydrate grams*
Crab (steamed)	93	93	3½ oz.	17	2	—
Eel (smoked)	330	190	2 oz.	11	17	—
Fish cakes						
fried	172	172	3½ oz.	15	8	9
frozen, fried, and reheated	270	270	3½ oz.	9	18	17
Fish sticks (frozen and cooked)	176	176	3½ oz.	17	9	7
Flounder						
baked	202	202	3½ oz.	30	8	—
Haddock						
fried	165	165	3½ oz.	20	6	6
smoked	103	103	3½ oz.	23	—	—
Halibut						
broiled	171	171	3½ oz.	25	7	—
smoked	224	224	3½ oz.	21	15	—
Herring						
kippered	211	211	3½ oz. 1 small	22	13	—
Lobster						
raw	91	91	3½ oz.	17	2	1
Newburg	194	194	3½ oz.	19	11	5
Mackerel (broiled with butter)	236	236	3½ oz.	22	16	—
Mussels (raw meat)	95	95	3½ oz.	14	2	3
Oysters (raw)	66	85	6 to 8 med.	10	2	4

Foods	*Calories in 100 grams**	*Calories per portion*	*Approximate size of portion*	*Protein grams*	*Fat grams*	*Carbohydrate grams*
Salmon, Atlantic						
broiled/baked	182	182	3½ oz.	27	7	—
smoked	176	176	3½ oz.	22	9	—
Sardines						
(canned)	203	203	3½ oz.	24	11	—
Scallops						
steamed	112	112	3½ oz.	23	1	—
frozen, breaded, and fried	194	194	3½ oz.	18	8	11
Shad						
(baked)	152	152	3½ oz.	15	9	2
Shrimp						
raw	91	91	3½ oz.	18	1	2
french fried	225	225	3½ oz.	20	11	10
Sturgeon						
(steamed)	160	160	3½ oz.	25	6	—
Swordfish						
(broiled)	174	174	3½ oz.	28	6	—
Trout, brook						
(raw)	101	101	3½ oz.	19	2	—
Tuna (canned)	197	197	3½ oz.	29	8	—

Meats and Poultry

Foods	*Calories in 100 grams**	*Calories per portion*	*Approximate size of portion*	*Protein grams*	*Fat grams*	*Carbohydrate grams*
Bacon						
(broiled/fried)	611	95	2 slices	5	9	1
Bacon						
Canadian (broiled/ fried)	277	85	2 slices	9	6	—

Foods	Calories in 100 grams*	Calories per portion	Approximate size of portion	Protein grams	Fat grams	Carbohydrate grams
Beef,						
chuck (braised/ roasted)	327	327	3½ oz.	26	24	—
loin or short loin (broiled)	465	465	3½ oz.	20	42	—
sirloin (broiled)	387	387	3½ oz.	23	32	—
rump (roasted)	347	347	3½ oz.	24	27	—
hamburger, regular (cooked)	286	286	3½ oz.	24	20	—
lean (cooked)	219	219	3½ oz.	27	11	—
corned beef (cooked)	372	372	3½ oz.	23	30	—
Chicken						
all classes						
light meat (roasted)	166	166	3½ oz.	32	3	—
dark meat (roasted)	176	176	3½ oz.	28	6	—
broilers (broiled)	136	136	3½ oz.	24	4	—
fryers (fried)	249	249	3½ oz.	31	12	3
roasters (roasted)	290	290	3½ oz.	25	20	—
Duck						
all parts (roasted)	326	326	3½ oz.	16	29	—
Goose						
all parts (roasted)	426	426	3½ oz.	24	36	—

Foods	*Calories in 100 grams**	*Calories per portion*	*Approximate size of portion*	*Protein grams*	*Fat grams*	*Carbohydrate grams*
Kidney						
beef (raw)	130	130	3½ oz.	15	7	1
calf (raw)	113	113	3½ oz.	17	5	—
lamb (raw)	105	105	3½ oz.	17	3	1
Lamb						
leg (roasted)	319	319	3½ oz.	17	21	—
loin chops (broiled)	420	420	3½ oz.	20	37	—
rib chops (broiled)	492	492	3½ oz.	17	47	—
shoulder (roasted)	374	374	3½ oz.	21	32	—
Liver						
beef (fried)	229	229	3½ oz.	26	11	5
calf (fried)	261	261	3½ oz.	30	13	4
chicken (simmered)	165	165	3½ oz.	27	4	3
lamb (broiled)	261	261	3½ oz.	32	12	3
Pork						
ham (roasted)	394	394	3½ oz.	22	33	—
ham cured (roasted)	310	310	3½ oz.	20	25	—
loin (roasted)	387	387	3½ oz.	24	32	—
spareribs (braised)	440	440	3½ oz.	21	39	—
Sausage						
bologna (fresh)	304	304	3½ oz.	12	28	1
frankfurters (raw)	309	309	3½ oz.	13	28	2
knackwurst (fresh)	278	278	3½ oz.	14	23	2
liverwurst (fresh)	307	307	3½ oz.	16	26	2

Foods	*Calories in 100 grams**	*Calories per portion*	*Approximate size of portion*	*Protein grams*	*Fat grams*	*Carbohydrate grams*
pork (raw)	498	498	3½ oz.	9	51	—
salami (dry)	450	450	3½ oz.	24	38	1
Sweetbreads						
calf (braised)	168	168	3½ oz.	33	3	—
Turkey						
light meat (roasted)	176	176	3½ oz.	33	4	—
dark meat (roasted)	203	203	3½ oz.	30	8	—
Tongue						
beef (braised)	244	244	3½ oz.	22	17	—
Veal						
loin (broiled)	234	234	3½ oz.	26	13	—
rib (roasted)	269	269	3½ oz.	27	17	—

Fruit

Foods	*Calories in 100 grams**	*Calories per portion*	*Approximate size of portion*	*Protein grams*	*Fat grams*	*Carbohydrate grams*
Apples						
fresh	58	70	1 med.	—	—	18
sauce (unsweetened)	91	100	1 cup	—	—	26
juice (bottled or fresh)	47	125	1 cup	—	—	31
Apricots						
fresh	51	20	1 med.	—	—	5
dried (uncooked)	260	220	½ cup	4	1	50
canned (in syrup)	85	220	1 cup	2	1	52
juice or nectar	57	140	1 cup	1	—	34
Avocado	167	185	½ large	2	19	7

Foods	*Calories in 100 grams**	*Calories per portion*	*Approximate size of portion*	*Protein grams*	*Fat grams*	*Carbohydrate grams*
Bananas	85	90	1 med.	1	—	22
Blackberries	58	85	1 cup	2	1	18
Blueberries	62	100	1 cup	1	1	23
Cantaloupe	30	45	½ med.	1	—	10
Cherries						
sweet						
(fresh)	70	75	1 cup	1	—	19
(canned)	81	200	1 cup	2	1	48
Cranberries						
fresh	46	53	1 cup	—	—	14
sauce						
(sweetened)	146	200	½ cup	—	—	50
juice	65	165	1 cup	—	—	55
Currants	54	38	½ cup	1	—	9
Dates, dried	274	100	3 or 4	1	—	26
Figs						
fresh	80	90	3 med.	2	1	22
dried	274	65	1 large	1	—	17
Fruit cocktail						
(canned)	76	195	1 cup	1	—	50
Gooseberries	39	40	1 cup	1	—	10
Grapefruit						
fresh	41	50	½ med.	1	—	14
canned						
(in syrup)	70	175	1 cup	2	—	42
juice						
(unsweetened)	41	100	1 cup	1	—	25
Grapes						
fresh	68	100	1 cup	2	1	24
juice	66	165	1 cup	1	—	41

Foods	Calories in 100 grams*	Calories per portion	Approximate size of portion	Protein grams	Fat grams	Carbohydrate grams
Lemon						
juice	25	4	1 tbs.	—	—	1
lemonade (diluted frozen concentrate)	44	110	1 cup	—	—	28
Olives						
ripe (Greek style)	338	235	10 large	2	25	6
green	116	75	10 large	1	8	1
Oranges						
fresh	45	60	1 med.	1	—	14
juice	45	110	1 cup	2	—	26
Peaches						
fresh	38	38	1 med.	1	—	9
canned	78	200	1 cup	1	—	50
Pears						
fresh	61	100	1 med.	1	1	25
canned	76	190	1 cup	1	1	48
Pineapples						
fresh	52	95	1 large slice	—	—	25
canned (heavy syrup)	74	185	1 cup	1	—	45
juice	54	130	1 cup	1	—	31
Plums						
fresh	66	30	1	—	—	7
canned	83	190	1 cup	1	—	48
Prunes						
cooked sweetened	180	450	1 cup	3	1	115

Foods	*Calories in 100 grams**	*Calories per portion*	*Approximate size of portion*	*Protein grams*	*Fat grams*	*Carbohydrate grams*
cooked						
unsweetened	119	300	1 cup	3	1	75
juice	77	190	1 cup	1	—	48
Raisins, dried	289	230	½ cup	2	1	62
Raspberries						
fresh						
(red)	57	57	¾ cup	1	—	13
(black)	73	73	¾ cup	2	1	16
Rhubarb						
(cooked						
sweetened)	141	380	1 cup	1	—	97
Strawberries	37	56	1 cup	1	1	12
Tangerines	46	35	1 med.	1	—	9
Watermelon	26	120	4″×8″ wedge	2	1	28
Nuts						
Almonds						
(roasted and						
salted)	627	180	1 oz.	5	16	6
Brazil nuts	654	185	1 oz.	4	17	3
Cashews	561	160	1 oz.	5	13	8
Hazelnuts	634	180	1 oz.	4	18	5
Macadamia nuts	691	195	1 oz.	2	20	5
Peanuts						
(roasted and						
salted)	585	165	1 oz.	7	14	5
Peanut butter	589	168	1 oz.	7	15	6
Pecans	687	195	1 oz.	3	20	4
Walnuts	640	180	1 oz.	4	18	5

Foods	*Calories in 100 grams**	*Calories per portion*	*Approximate size of portion*	*Protein grams*	*Fat grams*	*Carbohydrate grams*
Vegetables						
Artichokes						
Jerusalem						
(fresh)	7	7	1 large	2	—	—
(stored a long time)	75	75	1 large	2	—	17
Asparagus						
fresh (cooked)	20	20	6 to 9 spears	2	—	4
canned	21	21	4 large spears	2	—	3
Beans						
white (baked/pork and tomato)	122	244	¾ cup	12	6	38
kidney (canned)	90	230	1 cup	13	3	40
lima (boiled)	111	166	1 cup	11	1	30
green snap (boiled)	25	31	1 cup	2	—	6
Bean sprouts (boiled)	28	45	1 cup	5	—	7
Beets (boiled)	32	45	2, 2″ diameter	2	—	10
Broccoli (steamed)	26	40	1 cup	5	—	7
Brussels sprouts (boiled)	36	60	1 cup	7	—	9
Cabbage						
raw	24	28	1 cup	1	—	6
boiled	20	35	1 cup	2	—	7

Foods	*Calories in 100 grams**	*Calories per portion*	*Approximate size of portion*	*Protein grams*	*Fat grams*	*Carbohydrate grams*
Carrots						
raw	42	20	4 med. sticks	1	—	4
diced and boiled	31	45	1 cup	1	—	11
Cauliflower						
raw	27	16	2 oz.	2	—	3
cooked	22	30	1 cup	3	—	6
Celery						
raw	17	5	1 large stalk	—	—	1
cooked	14	14	1 cup	1	—	3
Corn						
boiled	91	91	1 ear	3	1	21
canned	84	170	1 cup	5	2	41
Cucumber (pared)	14	28	2 in.	1	—	6
Eggplant (boiled)	19	40	1 slice	2	—	8
Endive	20	9	2 oz.	1	—	2
Fennel	28	16	2 oz.	2	—	3
Leeks	52	10	1	1	—	2
Lettuce	15	15	¼ head	1	—	3
Mushrooms	28	28	6 med.	3	—	4
Onions						
raw	38	25	1 med.	1	—	6
boiled	29	70	1 cup	3	—	15
Parsnips (boiled)	66	100	1 cup	2	1	22
Peas (boiled)	71	71	1 cup	5	—	12

Foods	Calories in 100 grams*	Calories per portion	Approximate size of portion	Protein grams	Fat grams	Carbohydrate grams
Peppers						
sweet green (raw)	22	22	1 large	1	—	5
Pickles						
dill	11	4	1 oz.	—	—	1
sweet	146	42	1 oz.	—	—	10
Potatoes						
baked in skin	93	93	1 med.	3	—	21
french fried	274	165	12 pieces	3	8	22
mashed w/milk and butter	94	190	1 cup	4	9	25
chips	568	110	10 chips	1	8	10
sweet (baked in skin)	141	155	1 med.	2	1	36
Radishes	17	15	5 med.	1	—	3
Rice						
white (cooked)	109	185	1 cup	3	—	41
brown (cooked)	119	200	1 cup	4	1	45
Spinach (steamed)	23	23	1 cup	3	—	4
Squash						
summer (boiled)	14	38	1 cup	1	—	8
winter (mashed)	38	85	1 cup	2	1	18
Tomatoes						
fresh	22	33	1 med.	2	—	7
canned	21	50	1 cup	3	—	11
juice	19	50	1 cup	3	—	11
catsup	106	17	1 tbs.	—	—	4
Turnips (boiled)	23	40	1 cup	1	—	8
Watercress	19	10	1 cup	1	—	2

Foods	*Calories in 100 grams**	*Calories per portion*	*Approximate size of portion*	*Protein grams*	*Fat grams*	*Carbohydrate grams*

Cereal, Grains, and Breads

Foods	*Calories in 100 grams**	*Calories per portion*	*Approximate size of portion*	*Protein grams*	*Fat grams*	*Carbohydrate grams*
Biscuits	370	135	2½″ diameter	3	7	17
Bread						
white	270	61	1 slice	2	1	11
whole wheat	243	55	1 slice	2	1	11
rye	243	55	1 slice	2	—	12
corn bread	207	100	2″×2″ ×1″	3	4	15
Breakfast cereal						
bran flakes (40% Bran)	303	115	1 cup	4	—	30
cornflakes	386	110	1 cup	2	—	25
oatmeal (cooked)	55	140	1 cup	5	3	25
puffed rice	399	56	1 cup	1	—	12
shredded wheat	354	100	1 biscuit	3	1	22
Crackers						
graham	384	30	1	1	1	6
soda	439	25	1	1	1	4
Farina	371	400	1 cup	12	1	85
Flour (enriched, all-purpose)	364	400	1 cup	12	1	84
Macaroni (cooked firm)	148	200	1 cup	6	1	39
Macaroni and cheese (baked)	215	460	1 cup	18	24	44

Foods	*Calories in 100 grams**	*Calories per portion*	*Approximate size of portion*	*Protein grams*	*Fat grams*	*Carbohydrate grams*
Noodles (boiled)	125	200	1 cup	7	2	37
Pancakes	230	250	4, 4″ diameter	8	8	36
Pizza						
cheese and sausage)	235	175	⅛, 14″ diameter	6	7	23
Popcorn (oil and salt)	456	130	2 cups	2	6	17
Rice						
brown (uncooked)	360	750	1 cup	16	4	161
white (uncooked)	363	680	1 cup	13	1	154
Rolls						
Danish pastry	422	211	1 large	4	12	23
plain	312	120	1 med.	4	1	23
Spaghetti						
meat sauces	118	285	1 cup	13	10	35
tomato and cheese	90	230	1 cup	6	7	38
Waffles	275	210	1 med.	7	8	27

Soups

Foods	*Calories in 100 grams**	*Calories per portion*	*Approximate size of portion*	*Protein grams*	*Fat grams*	*Carbohydrate grams*
Thick (milk added, etc.)	85	210	1 cup	varies	varies	varies

Foods	*Calories in 100 grams**	*Calories per portion*	*Approximate size of portion*	*Protein grams*	*Fat grams*	*Carbohydrate grams*
Average thickness (meat and vegetables)	40	100	1 cup	varies	varies	varies
Light (bouillons, etc.)	13	32	1 cup	varies	varies	varies

Desserts and Sweets

Foods	*Calories in 100 grams**	*Calories per portion*	*Approximate size of portion*	*Protein grams*	*Fat grams*	*Carbohydrate grams*
Apple Brown Betty (crunch)	151	151	¾ cup	2	4	30
Bread pudding (with raisins)	187	375	¾ cup	6	6	28
Cake						
angel food	269	110	1 slice	3	1	24
chocolate (icing)	369	440	1 slice	5	20	67
fruitcake (dark)	379	115	2″×2″ ×½″	1	5	18
plain	364	200	1 slice	3	8	31
Candy						
butterscotch	397	112	1 oz.	—	1	27
caramels	399	112	1 oz.	1	3	22
chocolate (sweet)	528	156	1 oz.	2	10	15
chocolate (milk)	520	152	1 oz.	3	9	16

Foods	Calories in 100 grams*	Calories per portion	Approximate size of portion	Protein grams	Fat grams	Carbohydrate grams
chocolate-covered candies	410–570	117–163	1 oz.	2–16	11–44	40–81
fudge	400	114	1 oz.	1	3	21
hard (boiled)	386	111	1 oz.	—	—	28
Chewing gum	317	90	1 oz.	—	—	26
Chocolate syrup	330	120	3 tbs.	2	5	22
Cookies (assorted)	480	480	3½ oz.	51	2	71
Doughnuts (cake type)	391	130	1	2	6	17
Gelatin (with water)	59	236	1 cup	6	—	56
Honey (strained)	304	120	2 tbs.	—	—	33
Jams, jellies, preserves	273	55	1 tbs.	—	—	14
Molasses						
light	252	50	1 tbs.	—	—	13
blackstrap	213	45	1 tbs.	—	—	11
Pies (9″ diameter)						
apple	256	345	1/7th	3	15	51
blueberry	242	330	1/7th	3	15	47
cherry	211	350	1/7th	4	15	51
lemon meringue	255	300	1/7th	5	12	45
mince	271	365	1/7th	4	16	55
rhubarb	253	345	1/7th	4	14	52
Sugar (beet or cane)						

Foods	Calories in 100 grams*	Calories per portion	Approximate size of portion	Protein grams	Fat grams	Carbohydrate grams
granulated or powdered	385	18	1 tsp.	—	—	5
		385	½ cup	—	—	100
brown	373	410	½ cup	—	—	106
Syrup, maple	250	100	2 tbs.	—	—	25
Tapioca pudding	134	335	1 cup	13	13	43
Beverages						
Beer						
(4.5% alcohol by volume)	42	220	1 pt.	2	—	18
Gin, rum, vodka, whiskey (90 proof)	263	70	1 oz.	—	—	—
Wines						
dessert (18.8% vol.)	137	165	½ cup	—	—	9
table (12.2% vol.)	85	100	½ cup	—	—	5
Carbonated drinks						
soda (unsweetened)	0	0	12 oz.	—	—	—
quinine (sweetened)	31	107	12 oz.	—	—	28
colas (sweetened)	39	135	12 oz.	—	—	35
fruit-flavored	46	159	12 oz.	—	—	42
ginger ale	31	107	12 oz.	—	—	28
root beer	41	142	12 oz.	—	—	36
Coffee	1	0	1 cup	—	—	—
Tea	2	0	1 cup	—	—	—

APPENDIX 4

Specific and General Fitness Exercises for Men

The letters appearing after the name of each exercise indicate its primary or combined purposes:

(*st*) —stretching muscles
(*mu*) —muscle strengthening
(*ca*) —cardiovascular or general fitness exercises
* —This indicates the exercise will strengthen muscles if performed against resistance, like holding weights.

BACK EXERCISES

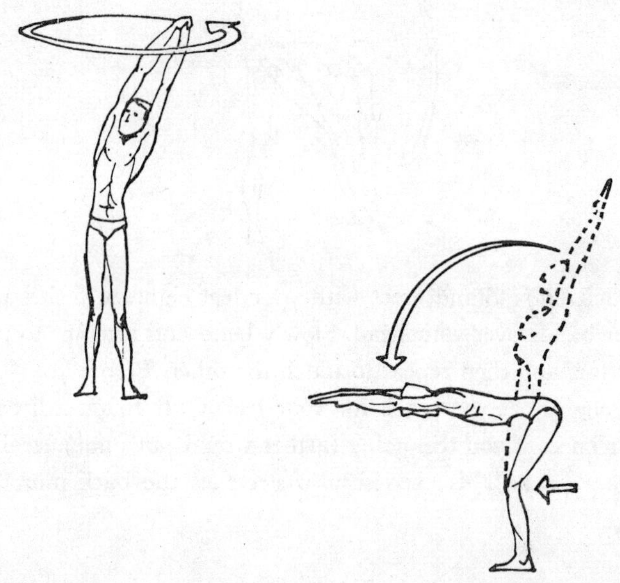

Circle Stretch (*st.*): (Above, left.) Keep your arms extended to their fullest and clasped over your head. Move them slowly in a large circle so that you feel all the muscles of your back, sides, and chest stretching.

Forward Stretch (*st, mu*): (Above, right.) Stand upright with your arms extended over your head. Suck in your stomach and slowly lean forward keeping your back straight until it's parallel with the ground. Allow your knees to bend a bit. Hold this position for two seconds. This is a difficult exercise and should be done with caution to avoid straining your back.

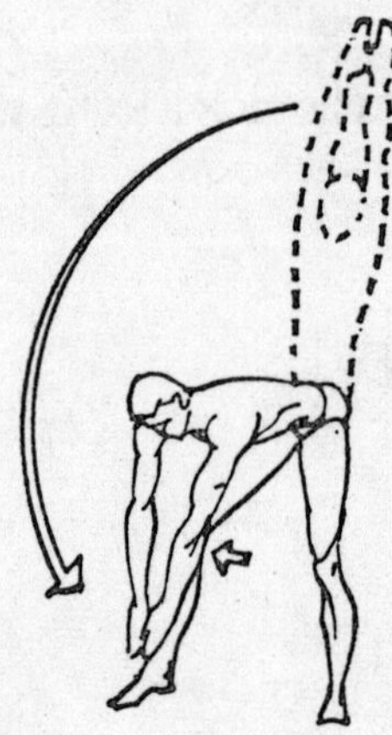

Toe Touch (*st*): Stand erect with your feet eighteen inches apart and your hands over your head. Slowly bend and attempt to touch first one toe, and then repeat to touch the other. Permit your knees to bend slightly as you reach for your feet. Only touch a little below your knees if you feel going farther would put undue strain on your lower back. This exercise also stretches the back muscles of your legs.

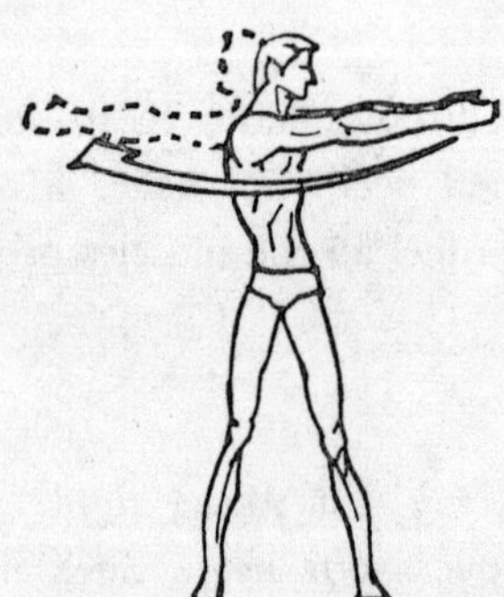

Body Twist (*st**): Stand erect with your feet eighteen inches apart and your arms extended parallel to each other and to the floor. Swing your arms in a continuous motion as far to the right and left as you can.

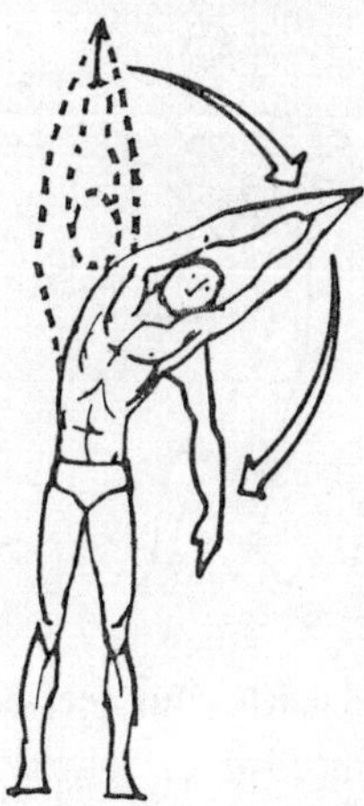

Side Stretch (*st**): Stand erect with your hands fully extended over your head and together. Slowly lean to the right as far as possible and then lower your right hand. You should feel all your side muscles stretching. Repeat the exercise on the left side. Holding weights will strengthen your waist and side muscles as well as your back.

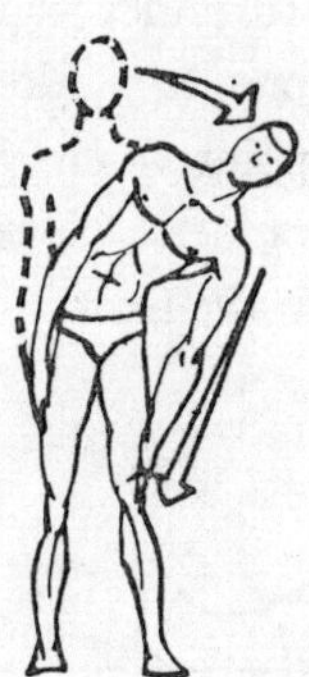

Side Lean (*st**): This is a milder form of the previous exercise. Stand erect with your arms to your sides. Lean to the right, extending your hand down your leg as far as possible. Repeat on the left side. This will build and stretch the muscles around your lower back.

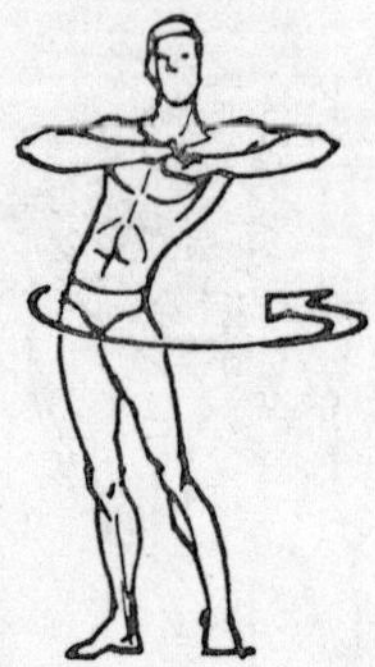

Hip Rotation (*st*): Stand with your feet eighteen inches apart and your hands either on your hips or joined at shoulder height with your elbows extended. Rotate your hips in an exaggerated circle so that you feel all your waist, side, and lower back muscles pull.

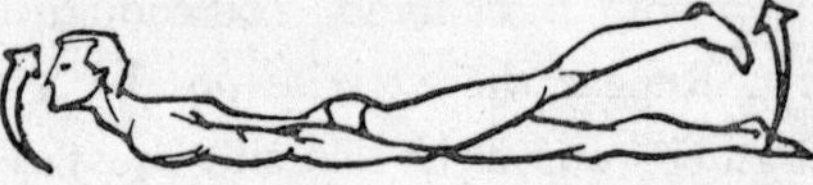

Spine Extension (*st, mu*): Lie face down on the floor with the palms of your hands upward under your thighs. Slowly raise your head and chest and lift one leg. Alternate with the other leg. Gradually progress to the point where you can lift both legs while raising your head and shoulders. Never lift your legs and chest more than a few inches from the floor.

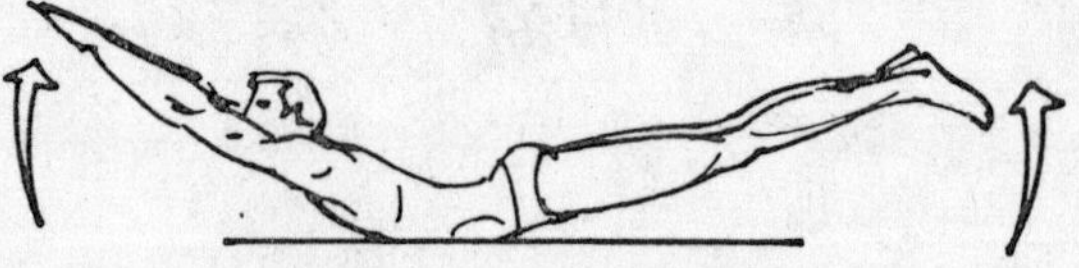

Spine Extension No. 2 (*st, mu*): This exercise is the same as the previous one except that your arms are extended ahead. This requires more effort. Do both spine extension exercises carefully, making sure not to lift your shoulders and feet too far off the floor.

SHOULDER, CHEST, AND ARM EXERCISES

Each of these exercises stretches and/or strengthens all three of these major muscle groups.

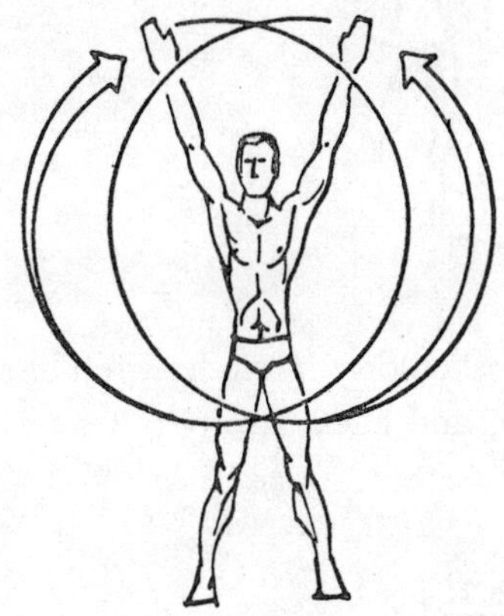

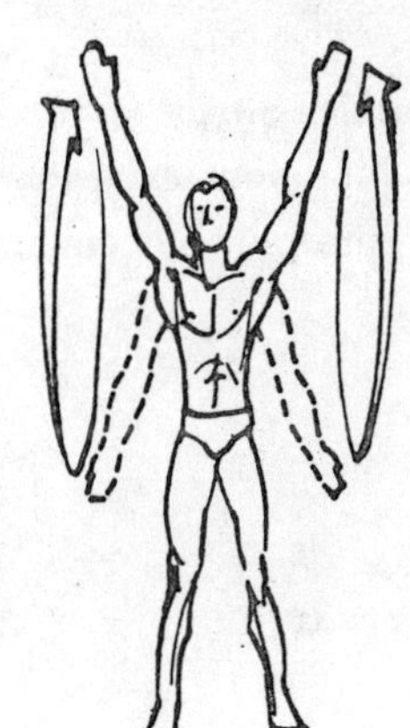

Cross Circles (*st**): (Above, left.) Stretch your arms to their limit and slowly move them in circles which overlap in front of your chest. You should feel all the muscles of your upper torso pull.

Side Circles (*st**): (Above, right.) Stretch your arms to their limit and slowly move them in circles at your sides.

Side Circle Twist (*st**) : While doing the previous exercise, slowly twist your arms from your wrists to your shoulders.

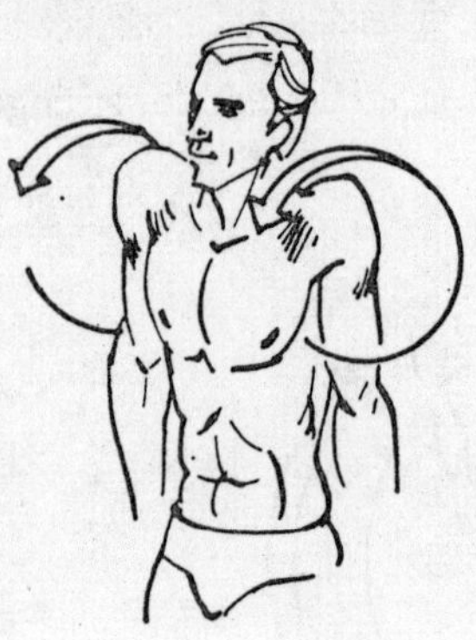

Shoulder Shrug (*st**) : Move your shoulders in circles from almost touching your ears, forward, down, and back. Really put some effort into your movements.

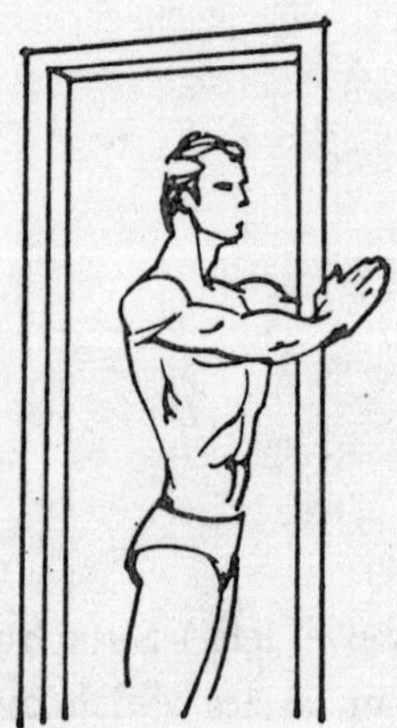

Chest Hold Isometric (*mu*) : Place the palms of your hands firmly on each side of a doorjamb with your elbows bent out. Press against the sides of the wall as hard as you can and hold. Stand upright with your lungs filled with air.

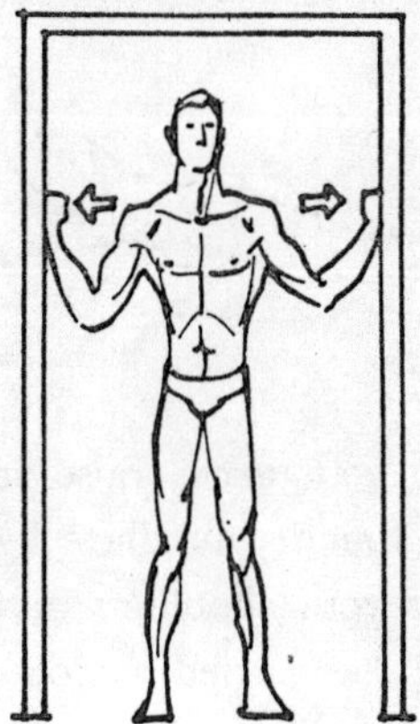

Shoulder Hold Isometric (*mu*): Place your palms firmly against each side of a doorjamb at shoulder height. Breathe in deeply and press outward with force. This exercise strengthens not only your shoulders but your upper back and arms.

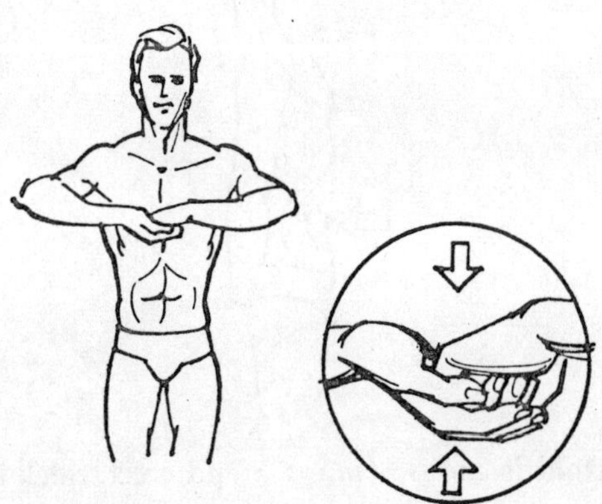

Fist to Palm Hold Isometric (*mu*): Stand erect, take a deep breath, and press the fist of one hand into the palm of the other, maintaining a strong static contraction. Alternate hands. This exercise should strengthen your front and rear arm muscles.

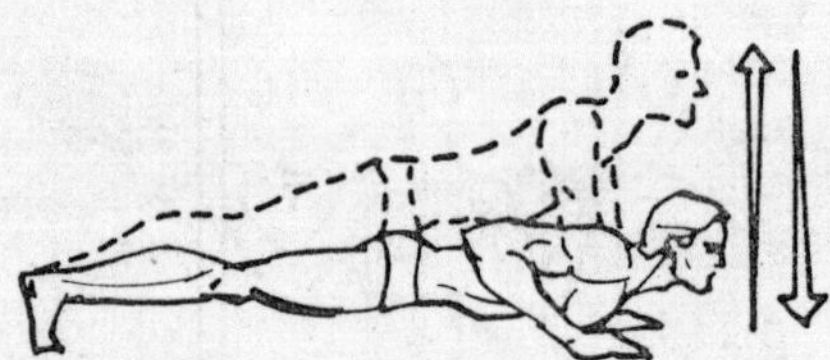

Press-up (*mu*): Using your arms, raise your body from a prone position and return to touch your chest lightly to the floor. Your palms should be under your shoulders and facing forward. Keep your back straight and toes curled as you do this exercise. It will build your upper body, shoulders, and arms.

ABDOMINAL EXERCISES

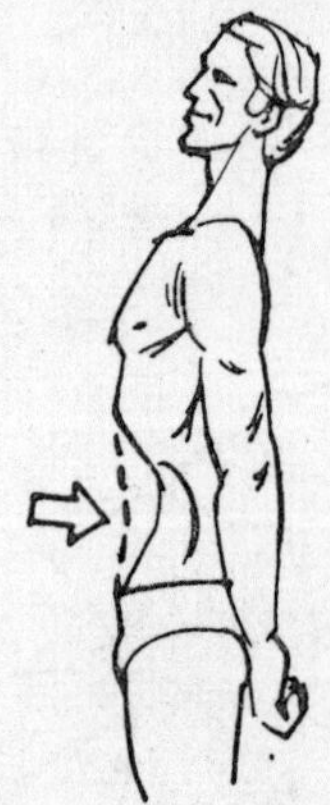

Abdominal Hold Isometric (*mu*): Stand erect. Suck in your stomach as hard as you can, using only your abdominal muscles. It should feel as if your stomach were pressing against your backbone. During the contraction, talk and breathe normally. Contractions of six seconds can be repeated with intervening relaxation. If you hold it for one minute, repeat it only two or three times a day with at least an hour's rest in between.

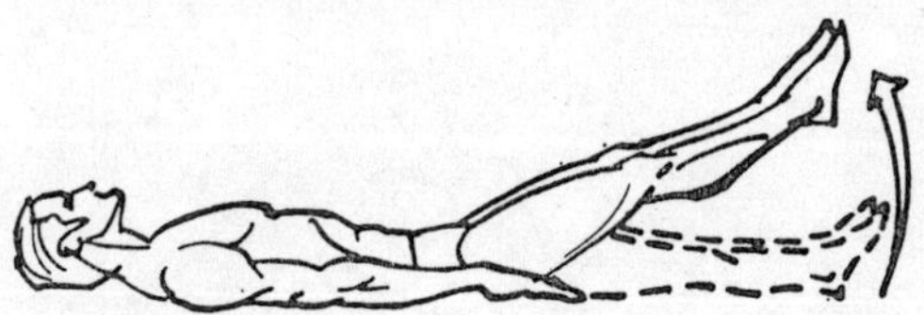

Leg Hold Isometric (*mu*): Lie on the floor with your lower back pressed to it and your arms by your side with palms down. Slowly lift both legs off the floor about twelve inches and hold that position for up to six seconds. Keep your legs stiff. This exercise also strengthens your leg muscles and back.

The following exercises from the posture section strengthen your abdominal muscles:

Half Sit-up
Knee Roll
Leg Roll
Leg Lift
The "U"

LEG EXERCISES

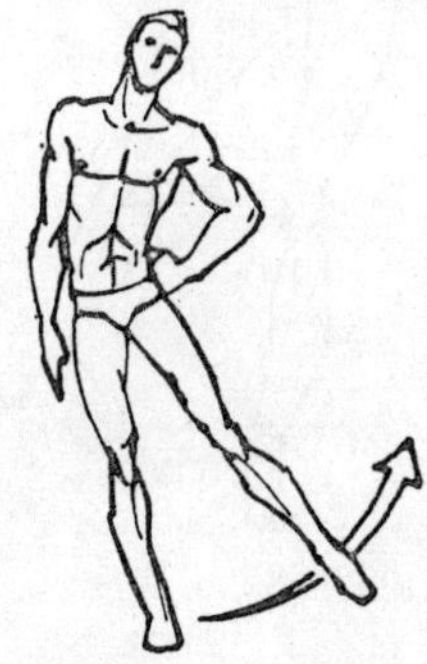

Leg Side Stretch (*st**): Stretch each leg to its limit while moving it up and out to the side. Contract your buttocks muscles while doing this exercise to firm them up.

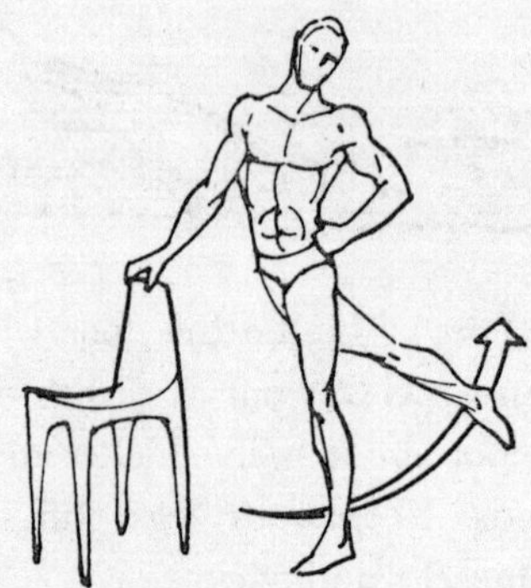

Leg Forward and Back Stretch (*st**): Stretch each leg to its limit and move it forward and back as far as you can. You may have to steady yourself by holding on to a chair. As with the previous exercise, contract your buttocks to strengthen and firm those muscles.

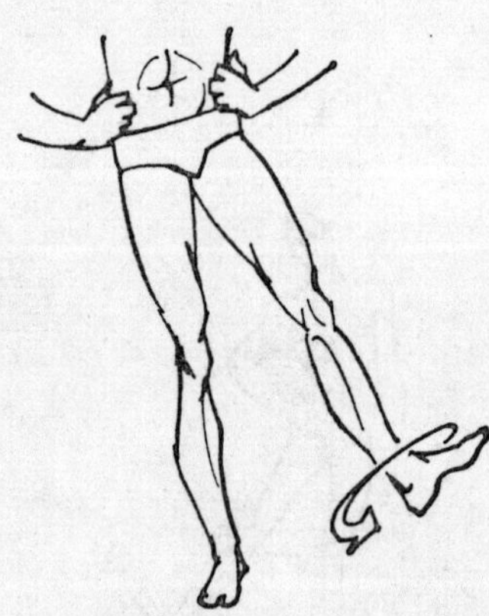

Ankle Twist (*st*): Extend your leg out and rotate your foot in all directions.

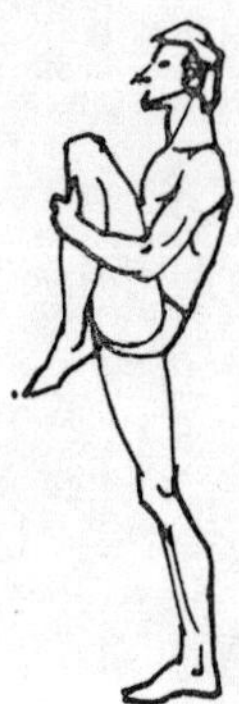

Knee Press—Upright (*st*): Balancing on one foot, press the other knee firmly to your chest. It may take time to work up to this one. Don't force things.

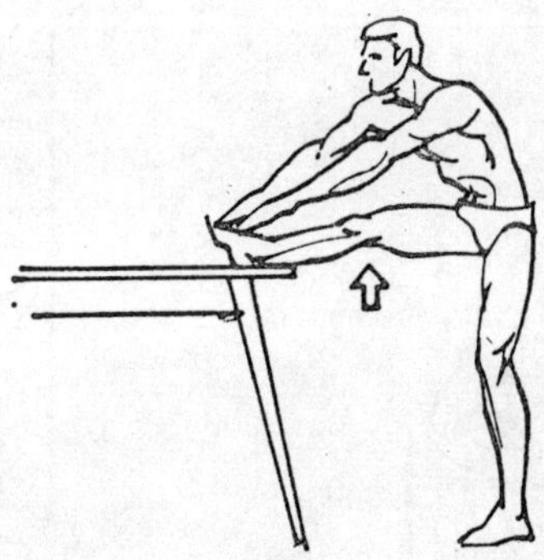

Hamstring Stretch (*st*): Place your foot on a table the same height as your hips and lean forward to touch your toes. Permit your knee to bend to relieve tension on your back. Don't strain yourself.

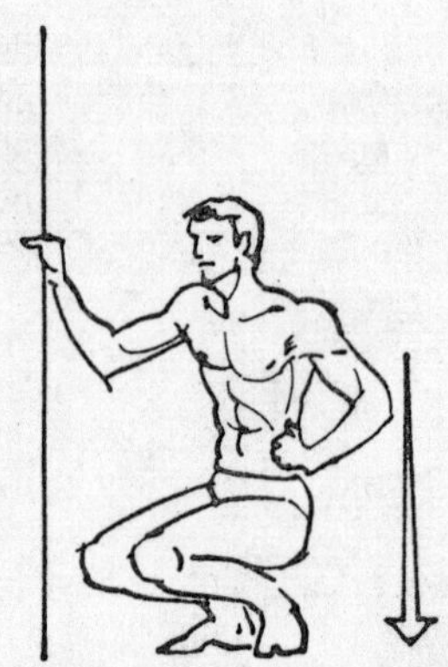

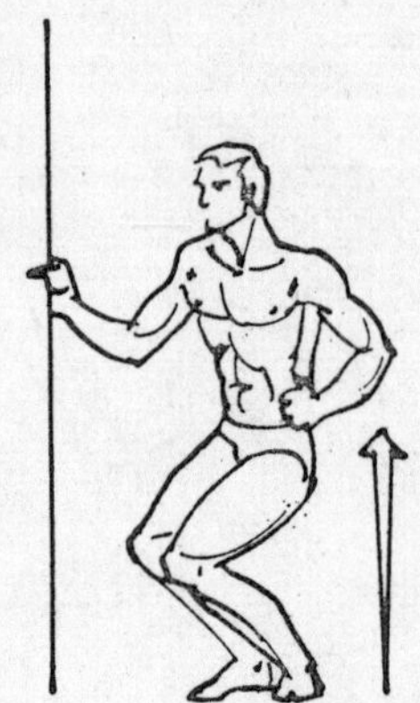

Knee Bend—Isometric/Isotonic (*mu*): Using a support, slowly lower yourself to a position where your buttocks are close to, but not touching, your heels. Hold this position for a few seconds while keeping your back upright. Raise up about one foot so that your knees are still bent. Hold that position for a few seconds. Repeat. This exercise can also be done in a continuing movement, which is easier, but not as effective.

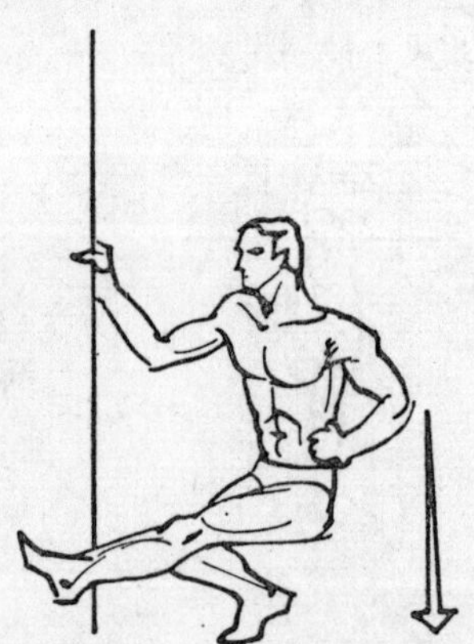

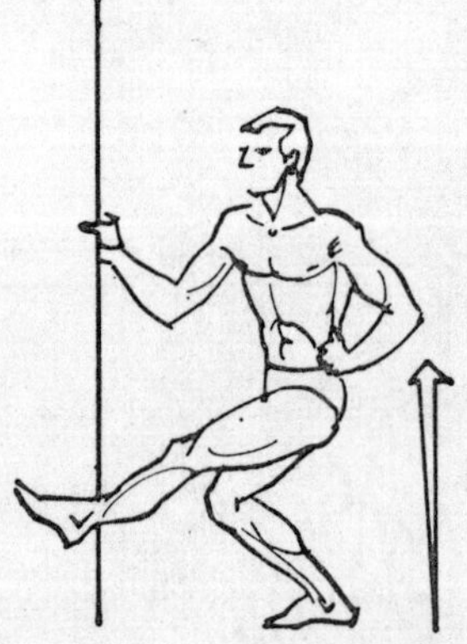

Knee Bend—Isometric Thigh Contraction (*mu*): Do the preceding exercise keeping one leg extended parallel to the floor. This is extremely difficult and should be done carfully so you don't strain your thigh muscles or back.

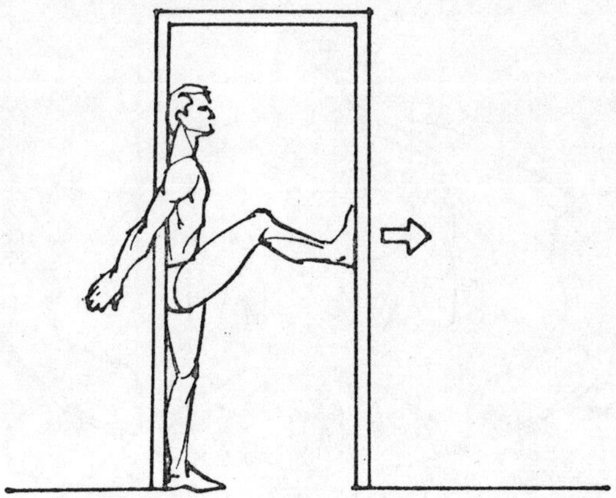

Door Press Isometric (*mu*): Place your head, shoulders, and lower back firmly against a doorjamb with your palm against the wall for balance. Press alternate feet against the opposite side at hip level and hold. This exercise strengthens the leg, hip, and stomach muscles.

NECK, CHIN, AND FACE EXERCISES

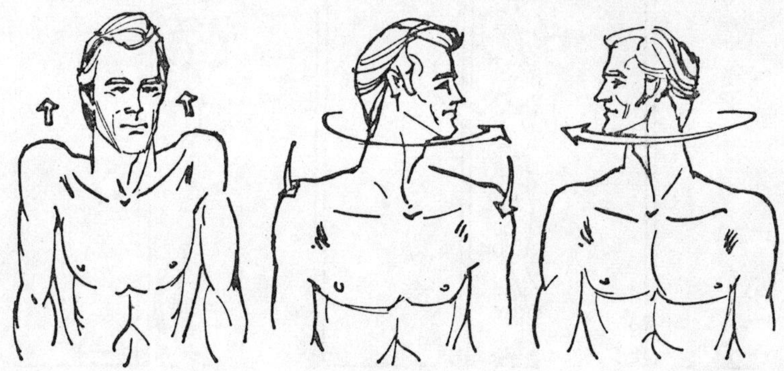

Over-the-shoulder (*st*): Lift your shoulders up to your ears and bring them all the way down. Then slowly turn your head to look as far over your right shoulder as you can and then rotate to look over your left shoulder.

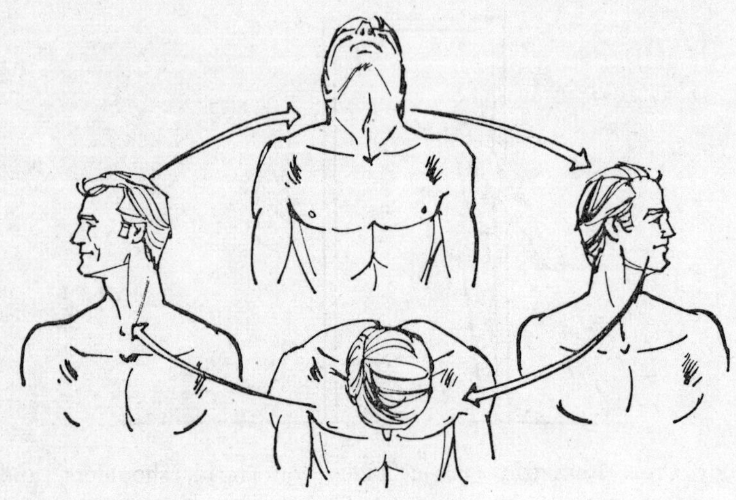

Head Rotation (*st*): Lift your shoulders up to your ears and then bring them down as far as possible. Extend your neck and slowly rotate your head in a circle from the chin touching your chest, to the side, head tilted back, and to the other side. Keep the movement smooth and feel your neck and shoulder muscles pull.

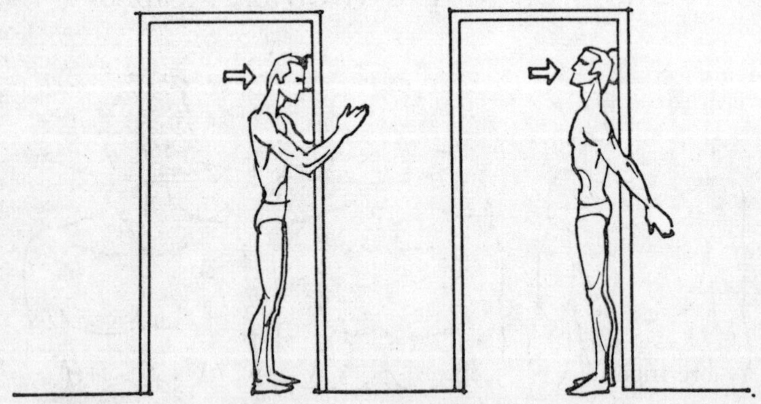

Neck Hold Isometric (*mu*): Place a pad between your forehead and a doorjamb. Stand straight with your hands holding the jamb. Press your forehead to the jamb and hold. This will strengthen your front neck muscles.

Reverse this position and lean back into the jamb to strengthen your back neck muscles. This exercise is valuable in relieving the symptoms of chronic neck strain.

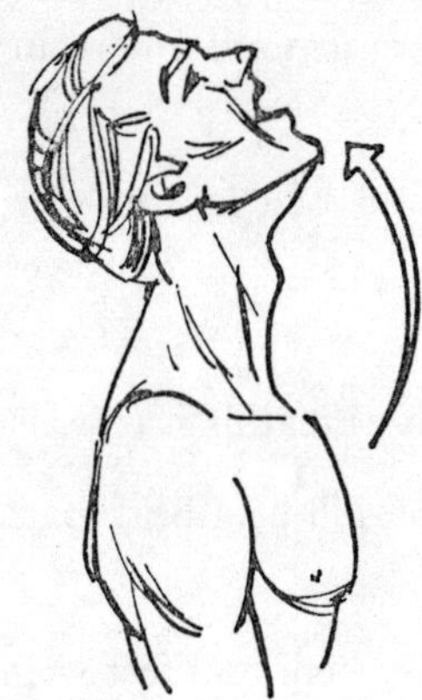

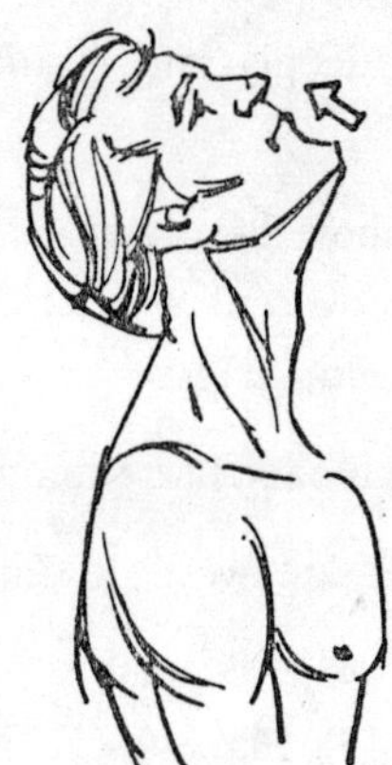

Chin Firmer (*st, mu*): Lift your shoulders up to your ears and then bring them down as far as possible. Open your mouth and tilt your head as far back as it will go. Slowly close your mouth, open it, close it. Repeat. You should feel a very strong pull against the muscles under your chin.

Face Contortions: The purpose of this exercise is to attempt to stretch every muscle in your face. In order to do this, you must distort your face so that you use muscles not normally used. Basically, the more frightful the faces you make, the better. Open and close your mouth while moving your jaw from right to left. Open and tightly shut your eyes, contracting your entire face at the same time. Try to touch your nose with your lower lip. Wink one eye after the other in rapid succession. *Warning:* Don't do this exercise in public or you may be locked away.

CARDIOVASCULAR AND GENERAL FITNESS EXERCISES

All of the exercises in this group involve dynamic movement and should be performed at a pace that makes you breathe hard. Breathe deeply and regularly. Don't overdo until you're in condition.

Active sport of any kind. Swimming is the best known exercise for the cardiovascular system. It involves the use of almost every muscle. (*st, mu, ca*)

Walk at a pace fast enough to cause heavy breathing. (*st, ca*)

Climb stairs two at a time or walk up a hill at a brisk pace. (*mu, ca*)

Running in Place (*ca*): Keep your knees high and feet well off the ground. Swing your arms and breathe deeply.

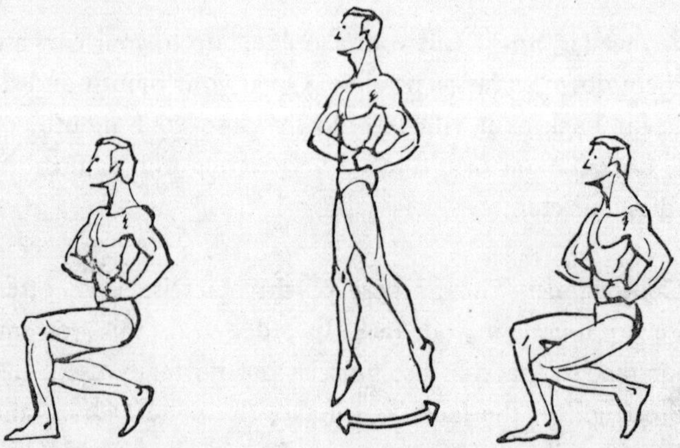

Squat Jumps (*mu, ca*): Stand upright with your hands on your hips. Jump up and come down into a squatting position with one foot in front of the other. Jump up again and come down with your feet in reversed positions. Do not come far enough down to touch the backs of your heels. Try to keep your back as upright as possible.

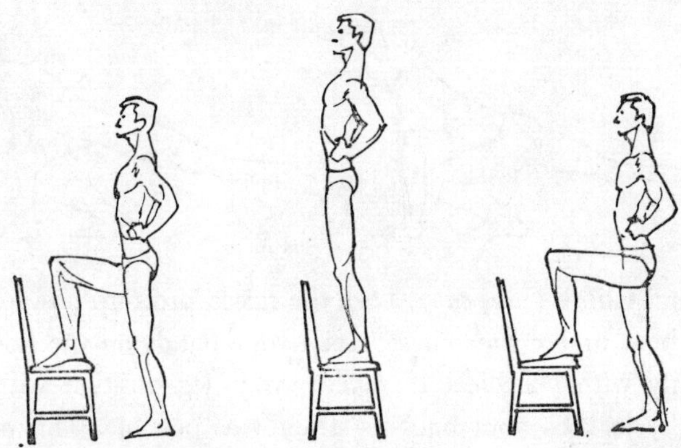

Chair Climbing (*mu, ca*): Stand in front of a chair (sturdy) or platform about twenty inches high. Place one foot on the chair, step up placing both feet on it, and step back down on the original foot. Keep your back straight at all times. Reverse your feet from time to time. One repetition should take about two seconds. This exercise is used to test one's endurance and fitness.

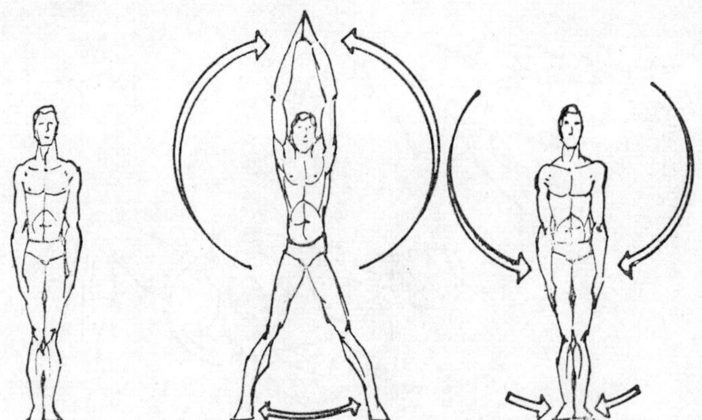

Windmill Jumps (*ca*): Stand at rest with your hands by your sides. Jump, swinging your arms over your head so your hands slap and come back to rest with your feet apart. Jump again, swinging your hands back down to your sides and bringing your feet together. Do this exercise in continuous, flowing movements.

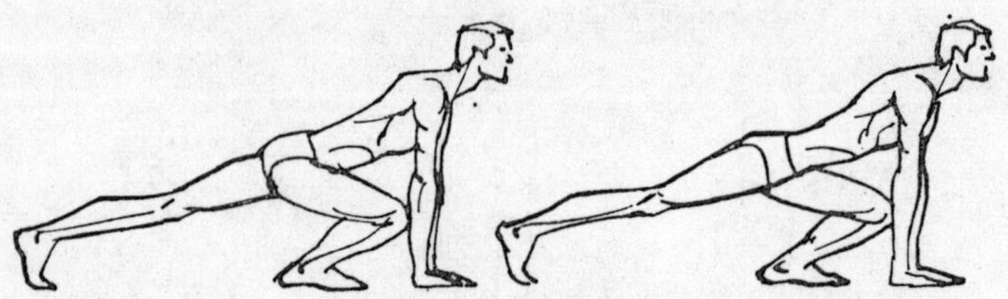

Horizontal Climb (*mu, ca*): Take the raised press-up position with one leg bent under your chest. Keep your hands on the floor and jump only with your feet to reverse your leg position with each jump. Try to keep your back as straight as possible. This exercise strengthens your legs, arms, shoulders, back, and midsection.

POSTURE EXERCISES

STRENGTHENING PROGRAM:

Pelvic Tilt—Vertical (*st*): Explained on page 221. Repeat up to twenty-five times.

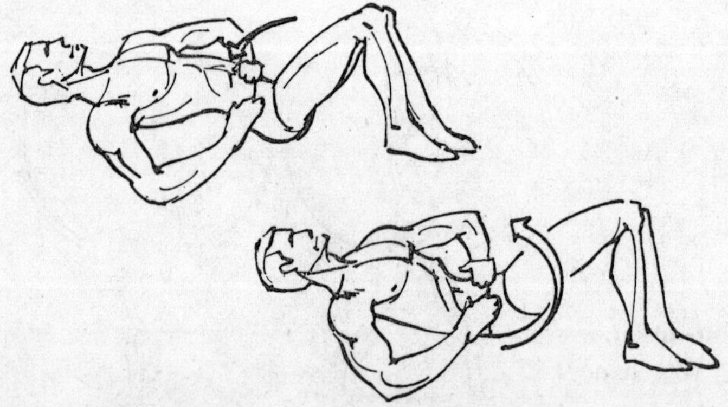

Pelvic Tilt—Horizontal (*st*): Lie on the floor with your knees bent and your hands on hips. Contract your buttocks and abdominal muscles while rotating or tilting your pelvis upward until the small of your back presses against the floor. Repeat up to 25 times.

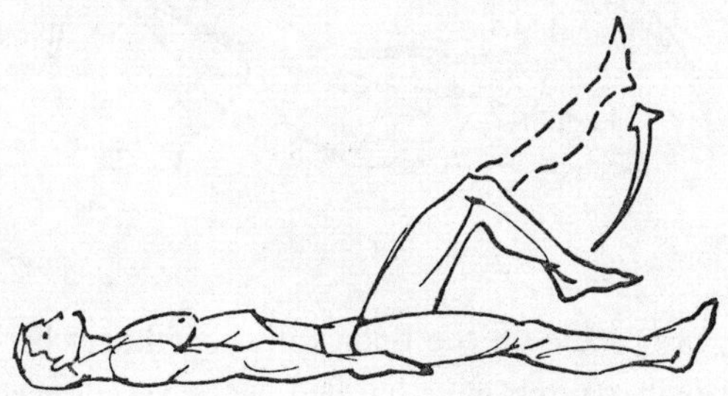

Leg Lift (*st, mu*): Lie on your back with your legs straight out. Start lifting one knee, and when it reaches a 45° angle with the floor, straighten your leg. Hold for a few seconds and then relax. Do with alternate legs. Repeat up to 25 times.

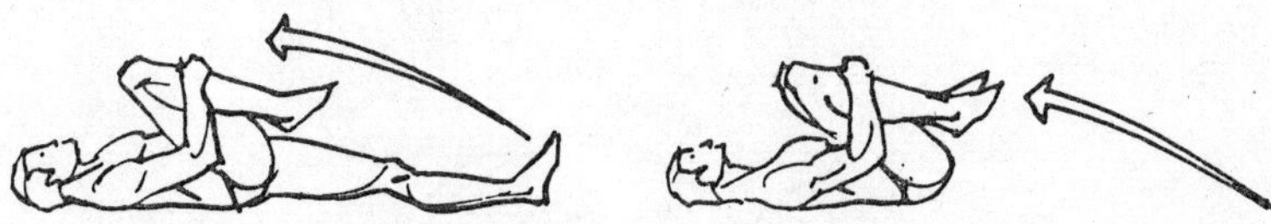

Knee Press—Horizontal (*st*): Lie on the floor with your legs straight out. Clasp alternate knees slowly to your chest. After ten repetitions, clasp both knees to your chest at the same time. Repeat 10 times.

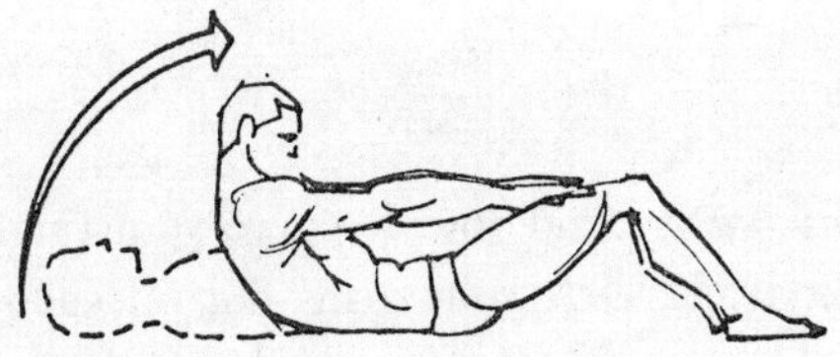

Half Sit-up (*st, mu*): Lie on the floor with your knees bent. Slowly stretch your hands toward your knees while rolling up the top part of your body (keeping your chin touching your chest). When the lower back is firmly pressing the floor, hold the position for three seconds and then relax. Repeat up to 25 times.

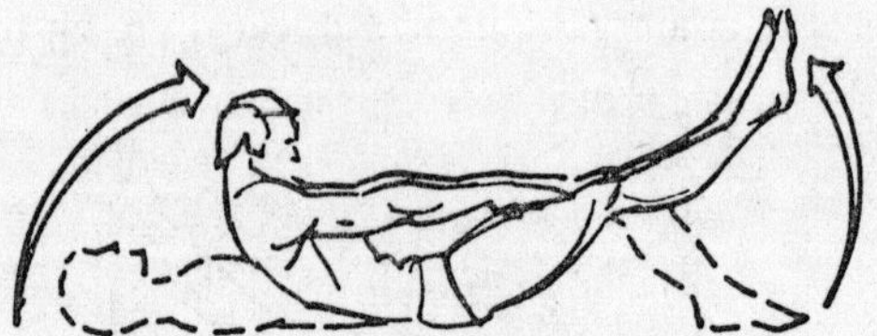

The "U" (*st, mu*) : Lie on the floor with your knees bent. Like the Half Sit-up, slowly stretch your hands toward your knees while you straighten your legs at a 45° angle with the floor. Touch your knees, hold the position for two seconds, then relax. Make sure the lower part of your body remains firmly pressed against the floor. Repeat up to 25 times.

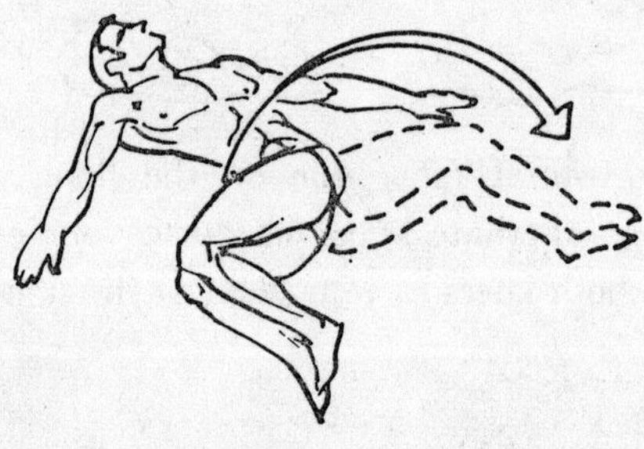

Knee Roll (*st, mu, ca*) : Bend your knees so your thighs are at right angles to your body. Stretch your arms out on each side, or hold on to something for support. Keep your shoulders firmly pressed to the floor. Keeping your knees together, slowly roll them to touch the floor on your right and then the floor on your left. Make sure the small of your back touches the floor when your knees are in the vertical position. Repeat up to 25 times on each side.

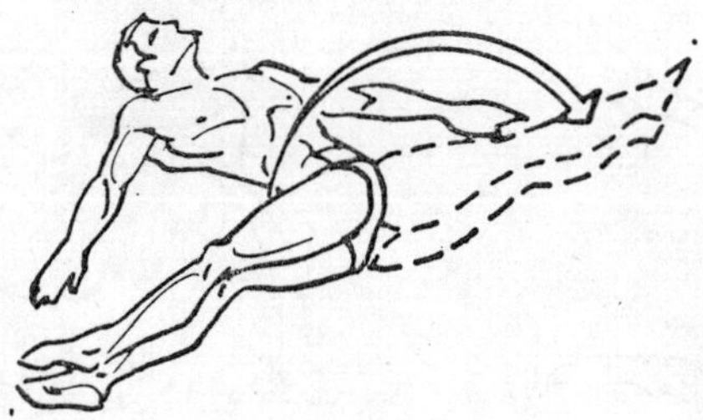

Leg Roll (*st, mu, ca*): This exercise is done in the same way you do the Knee Roll except that the legs are straight, not bent at any time. Try to keep your legs at right angles to your body. Repeat 10 times.

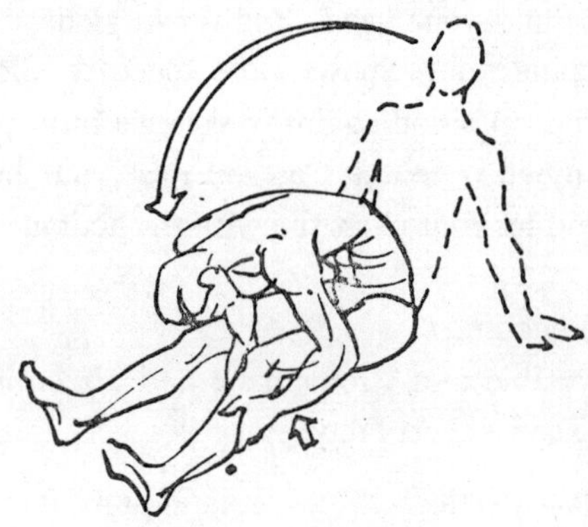

Forehead to Knees (*st*): Sit on the floor with your feet spread about eighteen inches apart and your back in a vertical position. Place both hands under alternate knees and try to touch your forehead to the knee, permitting the knee to bend. Do this exercise slowly and carefully and bend forward only as far as comfortable. Don't strain your back by overstretching. Eventually you may be able to complete this exercise without having to lift your knee from the floor. Repeat up to 10 times.

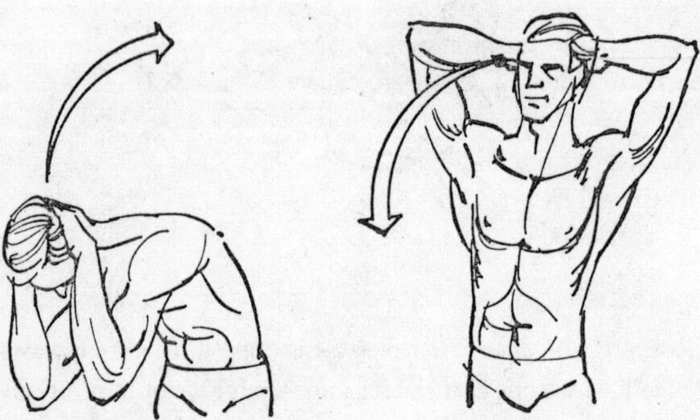

Neck and Shoulder Isometric (*st, mu*): Stand straight with your hands joined behind your head. Pull down against resistance from your neck, keeping your elbows close together. Slowly raise your head to an upright position against resistance from your arms. Your elbows should move wide apart as you raise your head. Keep your back straight and let your chest rise with the action.

MAINTENANCE PROGRAM

To maintain flexible and strong back and abdominal muscles, do the following exercises every day:

Pelvic Tilt—Vertical	25 repeats
Side Lean	25 repeats
The "U"	25 repeats
Knee Roll	25 repeats
or alternate with	
Leg Roll	10 repeats
or alternate with	
Forehead to Knees	10 repeats
Spine Extension No. 1 or No. 2	15 repeats
Neck and Shoulder Isometric	3 repeats, 6 seconds each

If you find you cannot manage the maintenance exercises comfortably, start gradually by doing the first four exercises in the posture strengthening program. As your fitness improves, increase the number of repetitions and then go on to the more difficult ones, culminating in the Forehead to Knees exercise. Always start off with Pelvic Tilts and Side Lean exercises to loosen up your muscles.

Bibliography

INGLIS, J. K. *A Textbook of Human Biology*. Pergamon Press, 1971.

HARE, P. J. "Your Skin," A Family Doctor Booklet. The British Medical Association.

———. *Basic Dermatology*. H. K. Lewis & Co., Ltd., 1966.

AVEDON, LUCIANA. *The Beautiful People's Beauty Book*. W. H. Allen, 1971.

KIBBE, CONSTANCE V. *Standard Textbook of Cosmetology*. Milady Publishing Corporation, 1972.

STABILE, TONI. *Cosmetics. The Great American Skin Game*. Ballantine Books, Inc., 1973.

* *

BATTLE, RICHARD. *Plastic Surgery*. Butterworths, 1964.

PERUTZ, KATHERIN. *Beyond the Looking Glass*. Penguin Books, 1972.

* *

FRYER, COLIN B. *Eye Health*. Gerald Duckworth & Co., Ltd., 1965.

* *

SCHERP, HENRY W. "Dental Caries: Prospects for Prevention." *Science*, Vol. 173, No. 4003 (September 24, 1971).

PADER, MORTON. "Dentifrices: Problems of Growth." Drug and Cosmetic Ind., June/July 1971.

FORREST, J. "Prevention in General Dental Practice—a Personal Philosophy." Gibbs Oral Hygiene Service.

CHALMERS, L. "Aspects of Dental and Oral Hygiene." S.P.C., November 1971.

BIBBY, BASIL. "Caries: Preventive Effects of Topical Fluoride Applications: A Review of Recent Clinical Trials in North America." *Bulletin of the Academy of Medicine of New Jersey,* Vol. 14, No. 4 (December 1968).

DUCKWORTH, ROY. "Review of Recent Clinical Trials Outside North America." *Bulletin of the Academy of Medicine of New Jersey,* Vol. 14, No. 4 (December 1968).

THOMAS, ADEEB, AND JAMISON, HOMER. "Effect of a Combination of Two Cariostatic Agents on Caries in Children: Two-Year Clinical Study of Supervised Brushing in Children's Homes." *Bulletin of the Academy of Medicine of New Jersey,* Vol. 14, No. 4 (December 1968).

MERGELE, MARVIN. "A Supervised Brushing Study in State Institution Schools." *Bulletin of the Academy of Medicine of New Jersey,* Vol. 14, No. 4 (December 1968).

———. "An Unsupervised Brushing Study on Subjects Residing in a Community with Fluoride in the Water." *Bulletin of the Academy of Medicine of New Jersey,* Vol. 14, No. 4 (December 1968).

VOLPE, ANTHONY. "Summary of Clinical Findings with a Monofluorophosphate Dentifrice." *Bulletin of the Academy of Medicine of New Jersey,* Vol. 14, No. 4 (December 1968).

* *

GODFREY, CORALIE. *Care of the Hands and Nails.* Saint Ann's Press, 1961.

* *

YUDKIN, JOHN. *This Slimming Business.* Penguin Books, 1971.

SOLOMON, NEIL. *The Truth About Weight Control.* Allen and Unwin, 1973.

WATT, BERNICE K., AND MERRILL, ANNABEL L. "Composition of Foods." U. S. Department of Agriculture.

MCCANCE, R. A., AND WIDDOWSON, E. M. "The Composition of Foods." Her Majesty's Stationery Office, 1969.

* *

AMELAR, RICHARD D. *Infertility in Men.* F. A. Davis Company, 1966.

SCHWARZ, OSWALD. *The Psychology of Sex.* Penguin Books, 1949.

CAUTHERY, P. *The Fundamentals of Sex.* W. H. Allen, 1971.

PEEL, JOHN, AND POTTS, MALCOM. *Textbook of Contraceptive Practice.* Cambridge University Press, 1969.

"Contraception: A Which? Supplement." 3d ed. London Consumers' Association, 1970.

"Methods of Birth Control in the United States." Planned Parenthood Federation of America, Inc.

"Basic of Birth Control." Planned Parenthood Federation of America, Inc.

LORAINE, JOHN A. "Endocrine Function in Subjects with Aberrant Sexual Behavior." *Steroids in Modern Medicine,* March 1972. Syntex Pharmaceuticals Ltd.

EISINGER, A. J., HUNTSMAN, R. G. AND LORD, JENNY. "Female Homosexuality." *Nature,* Vol. 328 (July 14, 1972).

* *

CATTERALL, R. D. *The Venereal Diseases.* Evans Brothers Ltd., 1967.

MORTON, R. S. *Venereal Diseases.* Penguin Books, 1970.

OWEN, ROBERT L., AND HILL, J. LAWRENCE. "Rectal and Pharyngeal Gonorrhea in Homosexual Men." *Journal of the American Medical Association,* Vol. 220 (June 5, 1972).

GUTHE, T., AND WILLCOX, R. R. "The International Incidence of Veneral Disease." *Royal Society of Health Journal,* Vol. 91, No. 3 (May/June 1971).

WILLCOX, R. R. "Perspectives in Venereology—1970." Bureau of Hygiene and Tropical Disease: *Abstracts on Hygiene,* Vol. 46, No. 10.

"V.D. Is One of the Facts of Life." Health Education Council.
"V.D., The Facts." Family Planning Association.

* *

MOREHOUSE, LAURENCE E., AND MILLER, AUGUSTUS T., JR. *Physiology of Exercise.* 6th ed. C. V. Mosby Company, 1971.

RANKIN, W. H. *Isometric Way to Instant Fitness.* Sphere, 1970.

WILLIAMS, J. G. P. "Posture and Physical Fitness." *Proceedings of the Royal Society of Medicine,* Vol. 62, No. 4 (April 1969).

Royal Canadian Air Force Exercise Plans for Physical Fitness. Pocket Books, Inc., 1962.

* *

NIXON, P. G. F. "Rehabilitation of the Coronary Patients." *Physiotheraphy.* 58, 10, 336 (1972).

———. "Recovery from Coronary Illness." Paper given to the 4th International Seminar on Rehabilitation, Edinburgh, June 29, 1971.

———. "The Prevention of Unnecessary Death from Coronary Heart Disease." *Health Visitor,* Vol. 43, November 1970.

———. "Exercise Therapy and the Coronary Patient." Presented at the Symposium on Testing in Rehabilitation in Cardiovascular Diseases, Bratislava, July 12, 1972.

NIXON, P. G. F., AND BETHELL, H. J. N. "A Myocardial Preinfarction Syndrome." *Medical World,* May 1972.

MACKINNON, ALISTAIR U. "The Psychopathology of Ischaemic Heart Disease." Paper read at Leeds General Infirmary at a refresher course in cardiology, January 28, 1967.

FREIDMAN, MEYER, ROSENMAN, RAY H. AND CARROLL, VERNICE. "Changes in the Serum Cholesterol and Blood Clotting Time in Men Subjected to Cyclic Variation of Occupational Stress." *Circulation,* Vol. 17 (May 1958).

CARNES, G. D. "Understanding the Cardiac Patient's Behavior." *American Journal of Nursing,* June 1971.

TREDGOLD, R. F. "Insecurity in Industry, Some Psychological Considerations." *Proceedings of the Royal Society of Medicine,* Vol. 65 (December 1972).

FROBERG, JAN, ET AL. "Conditions of Work: Psychological and Endocrine Stress Reactions." *Archives of Environmental Health,* Vol. 21 (December 1970).

PETER, LAURENCE J., AND HULL, RAYMOND. *The Peter Principle.* William Morrow & Company, Inc., 1969.

* *

OSWALD, IAN. *Sleep.* Penguin Books, 1970.

* *

FORT, JOEL. "Major Drugs: Their Use and Effects." *Playboy,* September 1972.

* *

MACFARLANE, SIR BURNET. *Genes, Dreams and Realities.* Medical and Technical Publishing Company, Ltd., 1971.

BROMLEY, D. B. *The Psychology of Human Aging.* Penguin Books, 1971.

GUNTRIP, HARRY. *Your Mind and Your Health.* Unwin Books, 1970.